Cardiovascular Physiology
A Text and E-Resource for Active Learning

T0143402

Cardiovascular Physiology
A Text and E-Resource for Active Learning

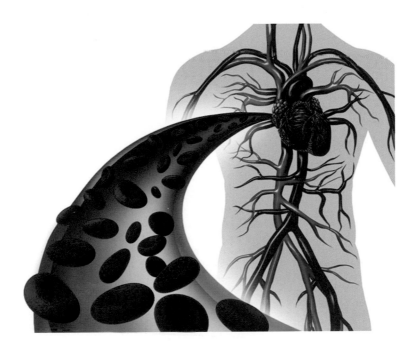

Burt B. Hamrell

Emeritus Professor, Department of Molecular Physiology and Biophysics,
College of Medicine, University of Vermont, Burlington, Vermont

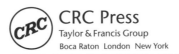

CRC Press
Taylor & Francis Group
Boca Raton London New York

CRC Press is an imprint of the
Taylor & Francis Group, an **informa** business

CRC Press
Taylor & Francis Group
6000 Broken Sound Parkway NW, Suite 300
Boca Raton, FL 33487-2742

© 2018 by Taylor & Francis Group, LLC
CRC Press is an imprint of Taylor & Francis Group, an Informa business

No claim to original U.S. Government works

Printed and bound in India by Replika Press Pvt. Ltd.

Printed on acid-free paper

International Standard Book Number-13: 978-1-138-09669-1 (Paperback)
978-1-138-09673-8 (Hardback)

Visit the Taylor & Francis Web site at
http://www.taylorandfrancis.com

and the CRC Press Web site at
http://www.crcpress.com

Contents

Preface   vii

Goals   ix

SECTION I   CARDIAC ELECTROPHYSIOLOGY AND THE ELECTROCARDIOGRAM (ECG)   1

1   Ventricular myocyte electrophysiology   3
    Resting potential   3
    Action potential   5
2   Cardiac electrical activity elsewhere than in ventricular muscle cells   9
    Sinoatrial (SA) node   9
    Atrial myocytes   11
    Atrioventricular (AV) node   12
    Bundle of His, bundle branches, and Purkinje myocytes   12
3   Physiological consequences of ionic mechanisms   15
    Pacemaker hierarchy and latent pacemakers   15
    Conduction velocity   16
    Refractory period   17
    Influence of extracellular K^+ concentration on the transmembrane potential (V_m) of ventricular and atrial myocytes   19
4   Control of heart rate   21
    Parasympathetic   21
    Sympathetic   21
5   Electrical properties and cardiac myocyte structure   23
6   Conduction of electrical activity in the heart   25
    Gap junction function   25
    Conduction sequence in the heart   25
7   Electrocardiogram   29
    Overview   29
    ECG waves   30
    Standard lead system   31
    Monitoring leads   35
    Frontal plane vectors   35
    Mean electrical axis   41
    Precordial leads   41
    ECG patterns of normal and abnormal heart conduction   42
    ECG patterns of abnormal rhythms: Arrhythmias   49
    Mechanisms of arrhythmias   52

SECTION II   CARDIOVASCULAR SYSTEM   59

8   How the circulation works   61
    Blood pressure   61
    Energy   61
    Flow   62

Contents

Blood flow types 64
Blood flow velocity in the circulation 67
Clinical significance 67

9   Cardiac cycle, heart sounds, and murmurs 71
The circulation 71
Cardiac valves 71
Atrial and ventricular phases of the cardiac cycle 71
Normal intravascular pressures in people 75
Heart sounds 75
Murmurs during the cardiac cycle 78

10   Ventricular function 83
Preload 83
Contractility 85
Afterload 88
Examples of changes in ventricular function 90
Ejection fraction 91
Passive (diastolic) pressure-volume relation 91
Control of the heart *in vivo*: A study summary 93

11   Peripheral circulation 95
Mean arterial pressure and pulse pressure 95
Resistance 100
Blood volume distribution 103

12   Circulatory controls 105
Introduction 105
Arterial neural baroreceptors 105
Hormonal controls 109
Chemoreceptors 116
Local metabolic control 116
Autoregulation 117
Arterial blood pressure and salt and water metabolism 119
Veins in circulatory control 119
Blood pressure control, the autonomic nervous system, and heart failure 120

13   Regional blood flow 121
Introduction 121
Cerebral blood flow 121
Coronary blood flow 124
Skeletal muscle blood flow 129
Pulmonary blood flow 130
Renal blood flow 132
Gastrointestinal blood flow 132
Cutaneous blood flow 132

14   Microcirculation 135
Arterioles 135
Capillaries 135
Metarterioles 135
Postcapillary resistance 136
Nature of blood flow in the microcirculation 136

References for additional reading 143
Index 145

Preface

The current emphasis in medical school teaching is on more active learning experiences in the basic sciences. Teachers are being asked to tell less and facilitate more active student learning. Students are being urged to reduce their expectation of being told what to learn and, instead, to learn how to learn. Hopefully, learning then becomes a lifelong skill. Patients rarely have symptoms and other findings as described in textbooks, they often respond differently than uniquely to treatment, and treatment and disease information changes continually. A competent physician cannot remain passive, but must actively pursue learning related to patient problems. The competent physician continually actively learns and thinks.

Teachers are being urged to enhance their skills developing goals and objectives and structuring student self-learning experiences. Student active learning source material often consists of traditional resources such as instructor's notes, textbooks or monographs, or current literature such as review articles. Used creatively, these materials can stimulate students to learn how to learn. However, the electronic self-study modules presented here are not the traditional material for discussion, but a learning resource that excites and engages the student learner. Today's student learners have grown up discovering information presented as electronic text, images, animations, and videos. Fortunately, contemporary cardiovascular medicine is awash with patient data presented as dynamic images, which can be configured, for instance, as animations that stimulate students to inform themselves and are optimally presented in an electronic format.

The electronic self-study modules presented here are active, self-learning, individually-paced experiences. The text that follows serves as a reference source for the self-study modules. The self-study modules include references to related parts of the text. The modules also include frequent opportunities to choose to review concepts. Study question sets are included for self assessment. The modules are designed to stimulate informal discussion among students and are a superb vehicle for stimulating discussion in small group sessions. I use them in this way in my teaching and they are uniformly successful.

The organization of the text and active learning modules follows the sequence of events in each heartbeat. The electrophysiological basis of activation of the heart and the heart's electrical activity as manifest in the electrocardiogram are presented first. Then the discussion proceeds to cardiac mechanical activity followed by the circulation of blood. The three-part self-study module on cardiac muscle mechanics should be studied before learning about ventricular function. Likewise, it is important to learn about the cardiac cycle early on since the terminology for describing pressures and flow is derived from the phases and events in the cardiac cycle.

The discussion of ventricular function precedes that of the peripheral circulation, circulatory controls, and regional circulations. The text concludes with a discussion of the microcirculation with emphasis on the dynamics of transcapillary fluid exchange and edema formation. The text also refers the reader to relevant self-study module presentations and, as noted above, each module cues the reader to relevant text material.

The self-study module on the pathophysiology of hypovolemic shock is included as a compelling emergency clinical problem, the discussion of which provides an excellent review of

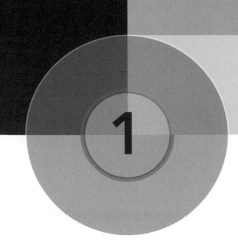

Ventricular myocyte electrophysiology

RESTING POTENTIAL

There are many positive and negative ions in the cell cytoplasm. Also, there are proteins in the cytoplasm with negative surface charges. Most of the positives and negatives interact as charge pairs to maintain electroneutrality. If every positive and negative ion were paired, the resting membrane potential would be zero. However, in resting ventricular muscle cells the electrical potential difference across the membrane, the resting transmembrane potential or resting potential, is about −80 to −90 mV (Figure 1.1). The negative sign indicates that the inside of the cell is negative with respect to the outside. The inside of the ventricular myocyte is negative mostly due to a *slight* deficit of potassium ions (K^+) inside the cell. This is because a small number of K^+ have left through open K^+ selective channels. Negative ions cannot accompany these K^+, leaving a small number of negative ions within the myocyte with no positive ion to associate with. Please note the emphasis on the word "slight." The key to understanding the genesis of a transmembrane potential is to realize that movement of very few ions across the sarcolemma is what is important; there is no measurable change in ion concentration inside or outside the myocyte. **This is presented with animations in the self-study module Cardiac Action Potentials, Part 1: Ventricular and Atrial.**

Charge separation by the sarcolemma with fewer positive than negative charges inside the cell can occur in the resting cardiac myocyte if two conditions are met:

- There are open sarcolemmal ion selective channels, the K1 channels, selective for K^+. These channels are neither voltage nor ligand gated, are continuously open, and can be called "leak" channels.
- There is a large K^+ concentration gradient with the K^+ concentration inside much higher than outside. A concentration *gradient* is critically important; a significant concentration *change* is not an important factor.

Since the K1 channels are selective for K^+, no ion can move with K^+ through the K1 channel. The K^+ moving out are attracted by the negative polarity of the cell interior and likely remain on the outside of the sarcolemma. Those negative ions inside the cell that lack a positive ion to associate with are attracted to the inside of the sarcolemma because of the positive exterior. Negative ions lining the inner surface of the sarcolemma and positive ions on the outer surface give rise to an electrical potential difference across the sarcolemma, the across-the-membrane or transmembrane potential.

The outward movement of K+ is opposed by the negative voltage that develops inside and the positive that develops outside the electrical gradient. That is why so few K+ leave the cell. K+ move out due to the concentration gradient and move in due to the electrical gradient. The concentration gradient is balanced by the electrical gradient at the K+ equilibrium potential, which is slightly more negative than the −80 to −90 mV resting potential in ventricular muscle cells. The K+ equilibrium potential is not reached because the sarcolemma is somewhat permeable to other ions, discussed below.

In healthy ventricular muscle cells bathed in an oxygenated interstitial fluid-like solution, the resting potential is stable (Figure 1.1, top graph, labeled 4) and does not change until an adequate electrical stimulus is applied to the muscle. **This is presented in the self-study modules Cardiac Action Potentials, Part 1: Ventricular and Atrial and Part 2: Nodal and Conduction System Myocytes.**

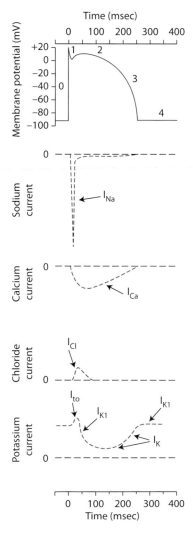

Figure 1.1 Ventricular action potential and ionic currents. (From Katz AM. *Physiology of the Heart*. 2nd ed. New York: Raven Press; 1992. With permission of Wolters Kluwer, Lippincott Williams & Wilkins.)

ACTION POTENTIAL

A ventricular muscle cell action potential develops in response to an adequate electrical stimulus. Adequate refers to an electrical stimulus that moves the transmembrane potential to a less
negative value, less negative than about -65 mV, where fast Na^+ channel external gates begin
to open. Once started, a ventricular action potential lasts roughly 250–300 ms—much longer
than a nerve or skeletal muscle action potential. The sequential portions of a cardiac muscle
action potential are labeled with numbers from 0 to 4 (Figure 1.1).

PHASE 0

Phase 0 is the initial rapid depolarization* or upstroke that occurs and initiates an action potential. As noted above, an adequate stimulus moves the resting potential to a less negative level
that triggers the opening of fast Na^+ channels. Ventricular muscle phase 0 is not substantially
different than depolarization in nerve and skeletal muscle.

An adequate stimulus causes voltage gated, ion selective fast Na^+ channels to open. The
Na^+ concentration is very low intracellularly, but is high in the extracellular fluid. The opening
of Na^+ selective channels leads to a rapid influx of a small number of Na^+ ions without accompanying negative ions. This large sodium current,† I_{Na}, rapidly depolarizes the cell (Figure 1.1).
The transmembrane voltage moves from negative to positive within 1–2 ms and reaches a peak
(Figure 1.1).

L-type Ca^{2+} channels are triggered to open during phase 0 when the transmembrane potential reaches -40 to -50 mV. These Ca^{2+} channels are slower to open and there are fewer of
them than fast Na^+ channels so their contribution to phase 0 is small. The Ca^{2+} current plays a
major role during phase 2, discussed below.

Depolarization stops at the peak of phase 0 at about $+20$ to $+30$ mV. Depolarization does
not reach the equilibrium potential for Na^+ (approximately $+70$ mV) because the Na^+ current
decreases and a K^+ current develops.

The Na^+ current decreases for two reasons:

- The inside of the cell becomes positive and this reduces the electrical potential driving
  force for the inward movement of Na^+.
- Depolarization rapidly inactivates Na^+ channels.

Both above factors contribute to a cessation of the voltage rise in phase 0.

A K^+ current develops for two reasons:

- The inside of a myocyte is positive with respect to the outside at the peak of the action
  potential. Like charges repel, so the inside positive "pushes" K^+ out of the cell.

---

* Depolarization indicates movement of the transmembrane potential in a positive direction; repolarization and hyperpolarization indicate movement in a negative direction.
† In the convention used by electrophysiologists, movement of positive ions into a cell is a negative current.
  That is why the Na^+ current in Figure 1.1 is shown moving downward. That can be confusing for other
  than an electrophysiologist, so I do not use the negative/positive current terminology. Simply read the
  graph for the sodium current as showing a rapid increase due to Na^+ moving inward followed by a rapid
  decrease as Na^+ channels deactivate. For the Ca^{2+} current there is a slow increase due to Ca^{2+} moving
  inward, then a slow decrease.

This alone would repolarize the membrane as I_{Na} decreases, but in addition,

- Phase 0 depolarization causes voltage-gated K^+ channels to open.

One such channel is the transiently outward or "to" channel. K^+ conductance transiently increases (Figure 1.1, bottom graph, I_{to}, a transient outward K^+ current). K^+ moving out of the cell is part of the reason phase 0 depolarization ceases at about +20 to +30 mV. I_{to} also contributes to repolarization in the next phase, phase 1. "K" channels are opened by phase 0 depolarization. "K" is the name of the channel and is not an abbreviation for potassium; K channels are distinct from the K1 channels. K channels are slow to organize and contribute little to the overall K^+ current until phases 2 and, particularly 3, discussed in more detail below.

PHASE 1

This is an initial repolarization following phase 0. It partially repolarizes the cell membrane from about +20 mV to just above 0 mV (Figure 1.1). This initial, brief repolarization is dependent on:

- Fast Na^+ channel inactivation.
- I_{to}, described above, an outward movement of K^+ ions through K_{to} channels.
- A small transient increase of Cl^- conductance triggered by depolarization. The extracellular concentration of Cl^- is much greater than inside the myocyte. Cl^- moves down its concentration gradient into the cell through briefly open ion selective Cl^- channels.

PHASE 2

After phase 1, repolarization slows dramatically to form phase 2, the *plateau phase* of the cardiac, action potential (Figure 1.1). It is a plateau, but not a perfectly flat plateau. During the plateau myocytes gradually repolarize for 100–200 ms. A plateau occurs primarily due to a partial balance of K^+ moving out of and Ca^{2+} moving into the myocyte (Figure 1.1).

I_{to}, a transient outward K^+ current, is important during phase 1, but the I_{to} channels deactivate early in phase 2 (Figure 1.1). The overall K^+ current decreases early in phase 2, but does not disappear. The reason that a small net K^+ current persists is related primarily to a persistent K1 channel current and a small contribution from the K channels.

K1 potassium channels, important for the resting potential, are rectified by depolarization. Rectification refers to a change in K1 channel function induced by depolarization such that K^+ ions do not as readily move through the K1 channels. The K1 channels are not closed, but are altered such that K^+ conductance is reduced. The decrease in overall K^+ current is due then to K_{to} channels deactivating and rectification of K1 channels (Figure 1.1).

Another reason the net K^+ current remains above zero during phase 2 is due to the slow (very slow) to activate K channels opened by depolarization during phase 0. Ventricular myocyte K channels consist of K_r and K_s components. Individual K_r and K_s components of the K channel current are not shown in Figure 1.1. The current due to the K channels takes a long time to become fully manifest. I_K does contribute in a small way to the net K^+ current during phase 2, but will play a key role during phase 3, when I_K is fully manifest. Remember, "K" here is not an abbreviation for potassium, but is the name of the channel.

As noted above, the L-type Ca^{2+} channels are voltage gated channels that open in response to depolarization to about −40 to −50 mV during phase 0. They begin to open during phase 0, but are slower to open than the fast Na^+ channels. I_{Ca} reaches a maximum early in the plateau and produces a depolarizing current. The presence of a net K^+ current pushes the transmembrane potential toward the negative. Ca^{2+} moving into the myocyte nudges the transmembrane potential toward the positive. The net effect of K^+ moving out and Ca^{2+} moving in is an almost steady transmembrane potential, the plateau. Inactivation of Ca^{2+} channels is slower than for Na^+ channels so the fall of the Ca^{2+} current is slow (Figure 1.1).

There is an electrogenic Na^+-Ca^{2+} exchange channel in the sarcolemma in which one Ca^{2+} moves out of the myocyte for 3 Na^+ in. That is three positive charges in for two out, three Na^+ in for one Ca^{2+} out. This is a depolarizing current. Ca^{2+} comes in through the L-type Ca^{2+} channels with each action potential so this exchange is important for preventing myocyte Ca^{2+} overload.

In summary, the ionic basis of the plateau is mostly explained by Ca^{2+} moving in and K^+ moving out. Some Na^+ ions move in as well.

The plateau portion of the ventricular action potential is important for two major reasons:

- Fast Na^+ channels remain inactivated during the plateau. The transmembrane potential during the plateau hovers at close to 0 mV. Na^+ channels remain inactivated at this transmembrane voltage and normally another action potential cannot be induced. This accounts for the long duration of refractoriness in ventricular myocytes. The long duration of refractoriness prevents extra depolarizations from occurring.
- Intracellular Ca^{2+} concentration increases. The small amount of Ca^{2+} that enters through the L-type sarcolemmal channels during the plateau triggers release of substantial amounts of Ca^{2+} from the terminal cisternae of the sarcoplasmic reticulum. This Ca^{2+}-induced-Ca^{2+}-release results in the large increase in cytoplasmic Ca^{2+} that initiates contraction. This small inward movement of Ca^{2+} and the significant increase in internal Ca^{2+} concentration due to Ca^{2+}-induced-Ca^{2+}-release is an exception to the rule that during an action potential there are no measurable changes in ionic concentrations.

As mentioned above, Ca^{2+} leaves the myocyte through a sarcolemmal Na^+-Ca^{2+} exchanger. Also, there is an active, ATP-energized pump that transports Ca^{2+} across the sarcolemma out of the myocyte. The net result of these processes is that a normal myocyte does not get overloaded with Ca^{2+}. The emphasis here is on "normal." Ca^{2+} overload can cause arrhythmias in heart disease and drug treatments and is covered in a later section on arrhythmias.

PHASE 3

The plateau ends and phase 3 begins with acceleration of repolarization (Figure 1.1). The return of the transmembrane potential from the plateau to the resting level is phase 3 (Figure 1.1, upper graph). Phase 3 repolarization is dependent on changes in K^+ and Ca^{2+} currents.

The overall K^+ current increases during phase 3 (Figure 1.1) as the I_K (K_r and K_s) channels reach full activation. I_K is the predominant repolarizing current. Congenital and acquired malfunction of the K_r or K_s channel is one cause of life-threatening arrhythmias or sudden death. One type of clinical problem is called the long QT syndrome and is discussed in a later section on arrhythmias.

During depolarization, rectification reduced the K1 current. Repolarization reverses rectification and K^+ movement through the K1 channels increases. I_{K1} then contributes to phase 3

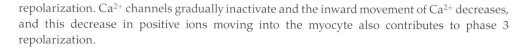
repolarization. Ca^{2+} channels gradually inactivate and the inward movement of Ca^{2+} decreases, and this decrease in positive ions moving into the myocyte also contributes to phase 3 repolarization.

PHASE 4

The interval between action potentials, when the membrane potential of a ventricular cell is at the resting potential, is called phase 4 (Figure 1.1). Phase 4 is stable in ventricular muscle cells due primarily to a stable I_{K1}.

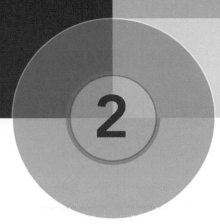

Cardiac electrical activity elsewhere than in ventricular muscle cells

To this point, only ventricular muscle cell action potentials have been discussed. But action potentials differ among the several types of heart muscle myocytes (Figure 2.1).

SINOATRIAL (SA) NODE

SA node cells depolarize in the interval between action potentials (Figure 2.2) and the most negative voltage level, the maximal diastolic potential (MDP), is −50 to −60 mV as compared with −80 to −90 mV in ventricular muscle cells. Diastole refers to the interval between heartbeats. The less negative level in SA node cells than in ventricular muscle cells is partly related to the limited expression of K1 channels in SA node cells.

Note the slow upward movement of the transmembrane potential during phase 4 from one bottom arrow to the next in Figure 2.2. This diastolic depolarization between action potentials during phase 4 is often termed the pacemaker potential. Diastolic depolarization during phase 4 brings the transmembrane potential to threshold and is responsible for repeated, rhythmic SA node cell action potentials.

The upstroke of the action potential during phase 0 is slow—the rate of rise of voltage relative to time, dV/dt, is slow (Figures 2.1 and 2.2). Additionally, the peak of phase 0 is at or slightly above 0 mV, not as high above zero as in ventricular myocytes.

PHASE 0 UPSTROKE (FIGURE 2.1)

Fast Na^+ channels that cause the rapid upstroke of a ventricular muscle action potential are either absent in SA node cells or not functional. Toward the end of diastolic depolarization (bottom right arrow in Figure 2.2), the transmembrane potential reaches the threshold for the opening of L-type Ca^{2+} channels. The current through these L-type Ca^{2+} channels, not Na^+ channels, produces depolarization during phase 0 in SA node cells. Phase 0 upstroke is slow with a small amplitude, because:

- L-type Ca^{2+} channels have slow kinetics.
- There are relatively few L-type Ca^{2+} channels in nodal cell sarcolemma.

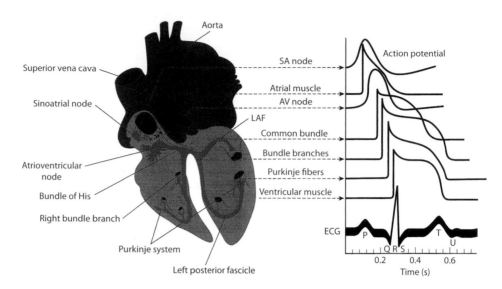

Figure 2.1 Action potentials throughout the heart. (Adapted from Barrett KE et al. *Ganong's Review of Medical Physiology*, 23rd ed. New York: McGraw-Hill; 2010. With permission of McGraw-Hill.)

PHASES 1 AND 2

There is no clearly identifiable phase 1 or phase 2 in an SA node action potential (Figures 2.1 and 2.2).

PHASE 3

K channels are important here just as in ventricular cells. Repolarization is due primarily to an increasing I_K and a decrease in $I_{Ca,L}$. The Ca^{2+} current decreases as Ca^{2+} channels deactivate. As noted above, the contribution from K1 channels is minimal. The transmembrane potential reaches the MDP primarily due to an increasing I_K and inactivation of $I_{Ca,L}$. Activation of I_f by repolarization, discussed below, contributes to MDP being less negative than in non-nodal cardiac myocytes.

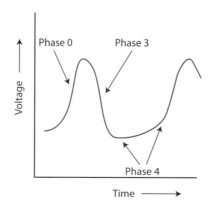

Figure 2.2 Sinoatrial node action potential. Diastolic depolarization (pacemaker potential) occurs during phase 4 between the two arrows. Phase 0 peaks at about zero volts.

PHASE 4

Four sarcolemmal ionic currents and intracellular Ca^{2+} cycling contribute to SA node diastolic depolarization during phase 4.

- I_f is a depolarizing current during phase 4. I_f channels support the slow movement inward of primarily Na^+. It is a peculiar ion channel ("f" stands for funny) in that it is activated by repolarization. Other voltage-gated channels are activated by depolarization. This channel also is referred to as the HCN channel: hyperpolarization-activated, cyclic nucleotide gated channel. As noted above, the onset of I_f at the end of phase 3 repolarization is one reason why the MDP is less negative than in non-nodal myocytes. Another reason is the minimal expression of K1 channels in nodal myocytes.
- Three Na^+/1 Ca^{2+} exchange (NCX) contributes to depolarization during phase 4 and NCX is related to cyclic changes in myocyte myoplasmic Ca^{2+} content. As noted above, phase 0 is due to the opening of L-type Ca^{2+} channels. The entry of Ca^{2+} into the cell initiates Ca^{2+}-induced-Ca^{2+}-release from the ryanodine-sensitive Ca^{2+}-release channels on the terminal cisternae of the sarcoplasmic reticulum (SR).

The increase in myoplasmic Ca^{2+} activates the Ca^{2+} pumps on the longitudinal portion of the SR. There is a Ca^{2+}-activated ATPase that hydrolyzes ATP and makes energy available to the pumps. These ATP-powered pumps move Ca^{2+} out of the myoplasm into the SR longitudinal tubules where the Ca^{2+} diffuses to and is stored at high concentrations in the terminal cisternae. **SR function is presented in more detail in the self-study module Clinical Heart Muscle Physiology, Part 1: Activation and Relaxation.**

Recent evidence indicates that in SA node cells, the terminal cisternae Ca^{2+} concentration reaches levels high enough to induce the spontaneous release of Ca^{2+} from them into the myoplasm. This localized Ca^{2+} release increases myoplasmic Ca^{2+} concentration.

The increase in intracellular Ca^{2+} and the low intracellular Na^+ concentration provide the driving forces for one Ca^{2+} moving out of the cell in exchange for three Na^+ moving in. Note: three positive charges (three Na^+) moving in and only two positive charges (one Ca^{2+}) moving out. 3 Na^+ in/1 Ca^{2+} out exchange produces a depolarizing current (I_{NCX}) including during phase 4. Localized Ca^{2+} release increases I_{NCX}, which contributes to diastolic depolarization.

- K channels open during phase 0 and I_K is important for repolarization during phase 3. I_K decreases during diastolic depolarization. This reduces the number of K^+ leaving the cell, positive charges stay in the cell, and this also supports phase 4 depolarization.
- $I_{Ca,T}$ involves Ca^{2+} movement through T-type Ca^{2+} channels. T-type Ca^{2+} channels open near the end of diastolic depolarization and contribute a brief, small depolarizing current. The T-type Ca^{2+} channels have a lower threshold and smaller conductance than L-type Ca^{2+} channels. "T" stands for tiny conductance and for transient.

Diastolic depolarization continues until it reaches the threshold for L-type Ca^{2+} channels and another heartbeat is initiated. **Nodal action potentials are presented in the self-study module Cardiac Action Potentials, Part 2: Nodal and Conduction System Myocytes.**

ATRIAL MYOCYTES

The resting potential is stable near -80 mV (Figure 2.1). Normally, there is no diastolic depolarization. Phase 0 has a rapid upstroke (Figure 2.1) and an overshoot (movement above zero), much as in ventricular cells. The upstroke is due primarily to the opening of fast Na^+ channels. The plateau slopes downward more than in a ventricular myocyte action potential (Figure 2.1) because of two factors. K^+ conductance during phase 2 and 3 is greater than in ventricular myocytes related to a more robust I_K. Also, there is a smaller Ca^{2+} current during phase 2.

The action potential is shorter than in ventricular or conduction system myocytes (Figure 2.1) related to a prominent I_K as noted above.

ATRIOVENTRICULAR (AV) NODE

The resting potential is slightly less negative (-60 to -40 mV) than in the SA node, but much less negative than in non-nodal heart tissue. Phase 4 depolarization is present, but is much slower than in the SA node. The mechanisms for slow diastolic depolarization are likely qualitatively like those in the SA node, but with much slower kinetics. The phase 0 upstroke and peak resemble the corresponding parts of the SA node action potential (Figures 2.1 and 2.2).

IONIC BASIS OF PHASES 0 AND 3

Fast Na^+ channels are absent or inactivated, like the SA node. The upstroke of the action potential is caused by the opening of L-type Ca^{2+} channels as in the SA node. Similarly, there is no identifiable phase 1 or 2. The mechanisms for phase 3 are like that in SA node cells.

PHASE 4 DEPOLARIZATION

The less negative resting potential than in ventricular myocytes and slow diastolic depolarization have mechanisms like those in the SA node. There are no likely major qualitative differences from the SA node. Quantitative differences in ionic currents result in much slower diastolic depolarization in AV node cells than in the SA node. The SA node is the normal pacemaker of the heart because its diastolic depolarization is faster than that of the AV node. This is discussed further below.

BUNDLE OF HIS, BUNDLE BRANCHES, AND PURKINJE MYOCYTES

PHASE 0

Phase 0 has a fast upstroke due to the opening of fast Na^+ channels that produce a large I_{Na}, just as in ventricular muscle. Note: even though Purkinje fibers have pacemaker activity, discussed below, they have an Na^+ action potential.

PHASES 1, 2, AND 3

The mechanisms for phases 1, 2, and 3 are like those in ventricular myocytes. Phase 1 is prominent and there is a long plateau (phase 2) (Figure 2.1).

RESTING POTENTIAL

His and bundle branch cells have stable K1 channel conductance during phase 4 and resemble atrial and ventricular cells in this respect. The resting potential is between -80 and -90 mV. The phase 4 transmembrane potential is stable in His and bundle branch fibers.

VERY SLOW DIASTOLIC DEPOLARIZATION IN PURKINJE MYOCYTES

Purkinje myocytes differ from other conduction system myocytes in that there is diastolic (phase 4) depolarization. The phase 4 diastolic depolarization is very slow. I_f channels are present and a slow increase in an Na^+ current through I_f channels contributes to the phase 4 depolarization. I_{NCX} and the opening of T-type Ca^{2+} channels also contribute to diastolic depolarization. T-type Ca^{2+} channels are not normally expressed elsewhere in the conduction system or in ventricular cells. The presence of K1 channels also influences the very slow diastolic depolarization in Purkinje myocytes. The movement of K^+ out of the cell through K1 channels is a repolarizing current that reduces the net depolarizing influence of I_f, I_{NCX}, and I_{Ca-T}.

The slight slope of phase 4 in a Purkinje myocyte action potential is not shown in Figure 3.1. Purkinje myocyte pacemaker activity can keep the ventricles beating, albeit at a very slow rate, if action potentials from the atria cannot get through to the ventricles (complete heart block, discussed later).

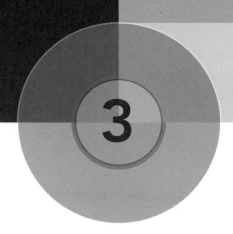

Physiological consequences of ionic mechanisms

3

PACEMAKER HIERARCHY AND LATENT PACEMAKERS

SA NODE

This is the normal pacemaker of the heart because diastolic depolarization is faster than in before AV node cells and much before Purkinje fibers **(self-study module Cardiac Action Potentials, Part 2: Nodal and Conduction System Myocytes)**. The pacemaker potential in SA node cells normally reaches threshold before the AV node cells and much before Purkinje fibers. The normal heart rhythm, driven by the SA node as the pacemaker, is called "normal sinus rhythm." The intrinsic frequency of the SA node, in the absence of input from the autonomic nervous system, is about 100 beats/min.

LATENT PACEMAKERS

AV NODE

Cells in the AV node can serve as the heart's pacemaker if, for instance, the SA node fails **(self-study module Cardiac Action Potentials, Part 2: Nodal and Conduction System Myocytes)**. The AV node intrinsic rate, i.e., with no autonomic nervous system input, is approximately 40–60 beats/min. If these cells become the pacemaker of the heart, the patient is said to be in atrioventricular junctional rhythm rather than normal sinus rhythm. "Junctional" refers to the pacemaker being at the junction of the atria with the ventricular septum. This rhythm can be diagnosed from an ECG. The AV node is innervated by sympathetic and parasympathetic nerve fibers, like the SA node.

PURKINJE FIBERS

The intrinsic frequency of Purkinje fibers is about 25–40/min **(self-study module Cardiac Action Potentials, Part 2: Nodal and Conduction System Myocytes)**. Purkinje fibers can become the ventricular pacemaker when there is complete failure of transmission of action potentials from the atria to the ventricles. The resulting abnormal heart rhythm is called complete heart block, complete atrioventricular block, or complete atrioventricular dissociation. In complete heart block, the ventricles regularly depolarize independent of the atria at the slow frequency likely set by a Purkinje fiber pacemaker and the atrial rate is separately set by the SA node.

CONDUCTION VELOCITY

DEFINITION

Conduction velocity is the time it takes for conduction of phase 0 from one point to another. Notice the emphasis on "phase 0." Conduction velocity has the usual units for velocity, distance/time, usually mm/ms.

DETERMINANTS OF CONDUCTION VELOCITY

RESISTANCE

A cell's internal resistance is inversely proportional to its diameter—the bigger the diameter, the lower the resistance. Cardiac cells are connected to each other at their ends. The larger the cell diameter, the lower the resistance, the faster the transmission of phase 0 along the length of the cell and, then, from cell to cell. Also, gap junctions lower cell-to-cell resistance and contribute to fast conduction. Gap junctions are non-selective ion channels embedded in the end-to-end connections of myocardial cells. They are discussed below.

PHASE 0 AMPLITUDE

A large amplitude phase 0 (again, notice the emphasis on phase 0) produces a large voltage difference between the cell being activated and the myocyte in phase 4 to which it is connected. A large amplitude phase 0 is based on movement inward of a larger number of Na^+ ions than when phase 0 amplitude is small. The probability of Na^+ ions passing to the next myocyte through the gap junctions is increased the more Na^+ ions enter during phase 0. Thus, the next myocyte will quickly depolarize to the fast Na^+ channel threshold. Similarly, Ca^{2+} moves from myocyte to myocyte through gap junctions in nodal tissues.

PHASE 0 dV/dt (VOLTAGE CHANGE PER UNIT TIME)

A fast upstroke rapidly depolarizes adjacent myocytes. In other words, a fast upstroke rapidly raises the transmembrane potential during phase 0 toward positive levels and rapidly increases the potential difference between depolarizing as compared with connected resting myocytes. The basis of a fast upstroke is the rapid movement inward of Na^+ ions. Myocytes that have a dense fast Na^+ channel population in their sarcolemma, such as in the conduction system, have a large dV/dt. Thus, Na^+ ions quickly reach the vicinity of the gap junctions and move through them to the next cell. A large dV/dt or fast upstroke during phase 0 is associated with fast cell-to-cell conduction.

CONDUCTION VELOCITY THROUGHOUT THE HEART

Note: Conduction velocity refers *only* to phase 0, the leading edge of the action potential, propagating from cell to cell.

- *His-Purkinje System*: In these large diameter cells with a fast phase 0 upstroke and large phase 0 amplitude, there is very rapid conduction (high conduction velocity), 1–4 mm/ms. Purkinje fiber phase 0 characteristics are related to the presence in the sarcolemma of a high density of fast Na^+ channels. Purkinje fibers have the fastest conduction velocity in the heart **(self-study module Cardiac Action Potentials, Part 2: Nodal and Conduction System Myocytes)**. Conduction velocity is influenced *only* by the characteristics of phase 0. Conduction velocity is not related in any way to phase 4 slow diastolic depolarization in the Purkinje fibers.

- *AV Node*: Most AV node cells a small diameter, a slow phase 0 upstroke, small phase 0 amplitude, and relatively few gap junctions **(self-study module Cardiac Action Potentials, Part 2: Nodal and Conduction System Myocytes)**. Therefore, conduction velocity is slow, roughly 0.05 mm/ms. The slowest conduction in the heart occurs here.
- *Atrial and Ventricular Muscle*: Intermediate cell diameter and phase 0 properties **(self-study module Cardiac Action Potentials, Part 1: Ventricular and Atrial)** result in intermediate conduction velocities of about 1 mm/ms. Conduction velocity is significantly less than in the conduction system.

REFRACTORY PERIOD

VENTRICULAR AND CONDUCTION SYSTEM MYOCYTES

ABSOLUTE REFRACTORY PERIOD (ARP)

In a normal ventricular myocyte, a stimulus cannot cause a conducted action potential during the ARP (Figure 3.1a). Ventricular myocyte Na^+ channels inactivate as the transmembrane potential approaches 0 volts during phase 0 **(self-study module Cardiac Action Potentials, Part 1: Ventricular and Atrial)**. Sustained depolarization during phase 2 keeps the Na^+ channels inactivated. The transmembrane potential must repolarize for the Na^+ channels to reactivate so that a stimulus will produce another conducted action potential.

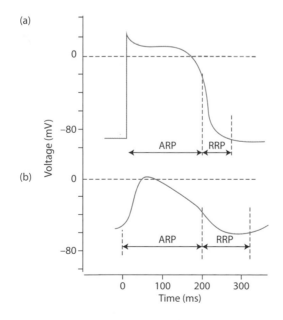

Figure 3.1 Refractory periods. **(a)** is a representative ventricular or conduction system myocyte action potential and **(b)** is a sinoatrial or atrioventricular node action potential. ARP is absolute refractory and RRP is relative refractory period.

The Na⁺ channels start to reactivate at the middle of phase 3, which is where the ARP ends (Figure 3.1a). Consequently, normal ventricular myocytes are refractory from phase 0, through the plateau to the middle of phase 3 (Figure 3.1a).

A long ARP in heart muscle cells is important to ensure that conduction proceeds only onward from myocyte-to-myocyte. If a myocyte did not become refractory with depolarization, the action potential, as it traveled from myocyte-to-myocyte, possibly could reverse direction, circle back to previously depolarized myocytes and induce aberrant action potentials.

Normal conduction in the heart starts at the SA node and proceeds only onward. Conduction normally never reverses direction. Refractoriness can become abbreviated, for instance, in damaged myocardium or resulting from drug effects. Conduction then can reverse direction and induce an extra action potential, something called reentry, and an abnormal heart rhythm (arrhythmia) is the result. Reentry is discussed later in the arrhythmia section of the discussion of the ECG (Section I, Chapter 7).

RELATIVE REFRACTORY PERIOD (RRP)

The ventricular myocyte RRP lasts from the middle of phase 3 to phase 4 (Figure 3.1a). During the brief RRP in ventricular muscle some Na⁺ channels are available to open whereas others have not yet recovered from inactivation. In the RRP a stronger than usual stimulus is needed to open enough Na⁺ channels to initiate a conducted action potential.

SA AND AV NODE REFRACTORY PERIOD

ARP AND RRP

Definitions of nodal myocyte ARP and RRP are the same as in the ventricle. Note that the combined ARP plus RRP extends well into phase 4 (**Figure 3.1b and self-study module Cardiac Action Potentials, Part 2: Nodal and Conduction System Myocytes**). The duration of ARP plus RRP, the total duration of refractoriness, in nodal cells is substantially longer than in ventricular muscle cells (Figure 3.1a and b). This is because Ca^{2+} channels, rather than Na⁺ channels, are responsible for depolarization of SA and AV nodal cells. All the Ca^{2+} channels must recover to restore full excitability of nodal cells. Ca^{2+} channel recovery kinetics are slow, so recovery of nodal cells takes a longer time than for the fast Na⁺ channels in non-nodal heart tissues.

PROTECTIVE FUNCTION OF LONG AV NODE REFRACTORINESS

An abnormally fast atrial rhythm can develop due to, for instance, disease or drug effects. Many of the atrial action potentials are likely to find the AV node refractory and do not propagate through the AV node into the conduction system. This can prevent a rapid abnormal atrial rhythm from inducing too rapid beating of the ventricles. Excessively rapid beating of the ventricles can limit the time available for ventricular filling and reduce cardiac output. This is an important clinical issue. Clinically, we think of the AV node as "protecting" the ventricles from beating too frequently with atrial tachyarrhythmias (fast abnormal atrial rhythms). The protective function of the atrioventricular node is related to its long total refractoriness. It is not related to and has nothing to do with the slow conduction through the atrioventricular node.

INFLUENCE OF EXTRACELLULAR K$^+$ CONCENTRATION ON THE TRANSMEMBRANE POTENTIAL (V$_m$) OF VENTRICULAR AND ATRIAL MYOCYTES

Resting V_m is strongly affected by the external K$^+$ concentration. The resting membrane potential becomes more positive (less negative; depolarized) if extracellular K$^+$ concentration is increased. This is because:

- K1 channels in resting ventricular, atrial, and conduction system myocytes remain open.
- An increase in external K$^+$ concentration reduces the concentration gradient across the membrane and movement of K$^+$ from inside to outside is hindered. The net effect is that more positive charges remain inside and the transmembrane potential shifts toward the positive. An equilibrium, where the concentration gradient is balanced by the electrical gradient, occurs at a less negative level. The greater the increase in external K$^+$ the more the cell will depolarize. **The pathophysiology of elevated serum K+ concentration, hyperkalemia, is discussed in the self-study module Cardiac Action Potentials, Part 1: Ventricular and Atrial**.

e

What is the likely effect on the resting transmembrane potential of a normal ventricular muscle cell if the extracellular Na$^+$ concentration is substantially increased?*

---

* The opportunity for Na$^+$ to enter a resting ventricular myocyte is extremely limited, so extracellular Na$^+$ concentration has virtually no effect on the resting transmembrane potential.

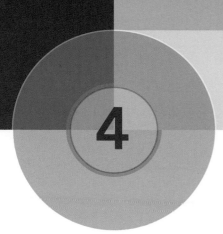

Control of heart rate

4

PARASYMPATHETIC

Acetylcholine (ACh) is the neurotransmitter released from postganglionic parasympathetic nerves ending on sinoatrial (SA) and atrioventricular (AV) node myocytes. There is some parasympathetic innervation of atrial myocytes, but sparse parasympathetic innervation of ventricular myocytes.

The chronotropic effect (effect on heart rate) of parasympathetic activity (Figure 4.1) is due to actions of ACh on SA node myocytes.

- ACh increases K^+ conductances and hyperpolarizes the maximum diastolic membrane potential during phase 4 (Figure 4.1).
- ACh also decreases the activation of I_f channels **(self-study module Cardiac Action Potentials, Part 2: Nodal and Conduction System Myocytes)** and because of this phase 4 depolarization starts from more negative levels, has a decreased slope, and takes longer to reach the threshold for initiating an action potential.
- Finally, ACh inhibits L-type Ca^{2+} channels, which slows the intracellular cycling of Ca^{2+}. The latter slows diastolic depolarization (Figure 4.1). The inhibition of L-type Ca^{2+} channels also raises the nodal action potential threshold.

The net result of the above is that diastolic depolarization starts from a more negative level, rises more slowly and must rise to a higher threshold to induce an action potential. This combination of effects results in a longer interval between beats and a reduced heart rate.

SYMPATHETIC

Norepinephrine is the sympathetic neurotransmitter and is released at sympathetic nerve endings on myocytes. Sympathetic nerves innervate all heart muscle cells. Also, sympathetic stimulation of the adrenal medulla results in the release of mostly epinephrine and some norepinephrine, which circulate as hormones and interact with cardiac myocytes.

Sympathetic stimulation of SA node cells increases the inward ionic currents of the pacemaker potential **(self-study module Cardiac Action Potentials, Part 2: Nodal and Conduction System Myocytes)** with a net effect of increasing the rate of diastolic depolarization (Figure 4.1). The effects are:

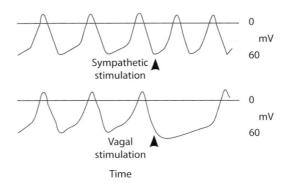

Figure 4.1 Effect of sympathetic and parasympathetic simulation on sinoatrial node action potentials. Note the threshold for the onset of phase 0 is lower with sympathetic stimulation and higher with vagal stimulation. (Modified from Barrett KE et al. *Ganong's Review of Medical Physiology*. 23rd ed. New York: McGraw-Hill; 2010. With permission of McGraw-Hill.)

- Enhanced opening of L-type Ca^{2+} and increased Ca^{2+}-induced-Ca^{2+}-release and an increase in I_{NCX}, a depolarizing current. The enhanced L-type Ca^{2+} channel opening lowers the threshold (Figure 4.1).
- Increased opening of I_f channels, which increases the slow inward movement of Na^+ and the slope of phase 4.

The combined effect of increases in I_{Ca}, I_{NCX}, and I_f **(self-study module Cardiac Action Potentials, Part 2: Nodal and Conduction System Myocytes)** are an increase in the upward slope of phase 4 (increased rate of diastolic depolarization) and a lower threshold for initiating phase 0 (Figure 4.1). Heart rate, as a result, increases.

- Sympathetic stimulation also enhances I_K, which accelerates phase 3 repolarization. A larger I_K would slow diastolic depolarization and heart rate, but the combined increases in I_{NCX} and I_f are enough to outweigh the enhanced I_K.

Electrical properties and cardiac myocyte structure

Cardiac muscle is partially composed of a highly branched network of small, 12 × 100 micron (μm) myocytes (Figure 5.1). There are several interchangeable names for a cardiac muscle cell: myocardial or cardiac muscle fiber and myocardial or cardiac myocyte.

Each myocyte is bounded longitudinally by intercalated discs and can branch (Figure 5.1). The intercalated discs connect myocytes end-to-end (Figure 5.1). Finger-like projections of the sarcolemma at the ends of myocytes are interlocked to form the intercalated disc. Desmosomes are dense areas of adherence within the intercalated disc (Figure 5.1). Desmosomes mechanically link myocytes and transmit force from one myocyte to the next. Of great importance are other specialized dense areas within the intercalated disc, the gap junctions (Figure 5.1),

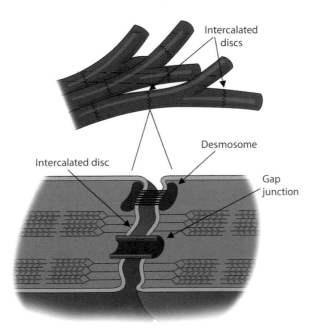

Figure 5.1 Intercalated discs, gap junctions, and desmosomes.

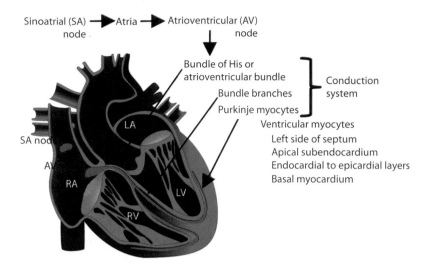

Sinoatrial (SA) node → Atria → Atrioventricular (AV) node

Bundle of His or atrioventricular bundle
Bundle branches
Purkinje myocytes
Conduction system

Ventricular myocytes
Left side of septum
Apical subendocardium
Endocardial to epicardial layers
Basal myocardium

LA

SA node

AV

RA

LV

RV

Figure 6.1 Sequence of electrical activation of the heart. RA, right atrium; LA, left atrium; RV, right ventricle; LV, left ventricle.

SINOATRIAL NODE

The sinoatrial (SA) node is in the right atrium at its juncture with the superior vena cava (Figure 6.1). The SA node is the normal pacemaker of the heart **(self-study module Cardiac Action Potentials, Part 2: Nodal and Conduction System Myocytes)**. As noted above, electrical activity begins here, initiates each heartbeat, and then spreads throughout the atria.

ATRIAL MUSCLE

Electrical activity is conducted from atrial myocyte to atrial myocyte throughout the right and left atria primarily via gap junctions.

ATRIOVENTRICULAR NODE

The AV node is in the right atrium at the bottom of the interatrial septum near the opening of the coronary sinus. It conducts electrical activity from the atria to the bundle of His (Figure 6.1). Electrical conduction in the AV node, as noted earlier, is very slow.

Slow AV nodal conduction is important. Slow conduction ensures that atrial activation and contraction are completed before ventricular activation and contraction begin. Atrial contraction then will occur when the ventricles are still relaxed.

There is a connective tissue structure, the annulus fibrosus (Figure 6.2), that electrically insulates the atria from the ventricles. The bundle of His or atrioventricular bundle (Figures 6.1 and 6.2), discussed below, penetrates the annulus. The only normal pathway for conduction of action potentials from the atria to the ventricles begins in the AV nodal tissue and then continues in the cardiac myocytes of the bundle of His through the connective tissue electrical barrier (Figure 6.2).

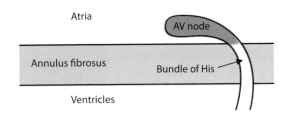

Figure 6.2 Atrioventricular node, annulus fibrosus, and the bundle of His.

VENTRICULAR CONDUCTION SYSTEM

The ventricular conducting system consists of the bundle of His or atrioventricular bundle, the bundle branches, and the Purkinje system (Figure 6.1). The AV node merges with the bundle of His (Figure 6.2), but is not considered part of the conduction system.

At the top of the interventricular septum, the bundle of His divides into the left and right bundle branches (Figure 6.1) that distribute action potentials to the left and right ventricles, respectively. The bundle branches continue to branch extensively in the subendocardial layers of both ventricles. The Purkinje myocytes are the terminal branches of the conduction system (Figure 6.1).

The conduction system is not nerve tissue. It is made up of myocytes, but they are specialized for rapid conduction **(self-study module Cardiac Action Potentials, Part 2: Nodal and Conduction System Myocytes)**. Purkinje myocytes contain large amounts of glycogen and are resistant to hypoxia.

The His bundle and bundle branches are surrounded by connective tissue sheaths. The connective tissue sheath insulates these conduction system cells from the surrounding ventricular muscle. Therefore, the first electrical contact with ventricular myocytes is not made until the Purkinje myocytes merge into ventricular myocytes. Purkinje fibers do not have connective tissue sheaths.

The sequence of normal ventricular activation (Figure 6.1):

- Left side of the ventricular septum is first, followed by
- Subendocardial myocardium of ventricular apex, then
- Subendocardial myocardium of the ventricles, then
- From inner subendocardial layers out to subepicardial myocardium, and
- Simultaneously from apex to base—left and right ventricular bases are last

Activation proceeds from endocardial, inner layers of the ventricular wall to the outer, subepicardial layers and from the apex of the ventricles toward the base of each ventricle. The ventricular myocardium attached to the annulus fibrosus is the base. The bases of the right and left ventricles depolarize last. The last location to depolarize usually is the outflow tract of the right ventricle, just proximal to the pulmonary valve.

ECG WAVES

During a heartbeat, a series of voltage deflections or waves are recorded. Einthoven named these the P wave, a sequence of waves called the QRS complex, and the T wave. There are also intervals and segments. An interval includes at least one wave whereas a segment does not include a wave.

P WAVE

The P wave (Figure 7.1) is the body surface recording of the sequential depolarization (phase 0) of atrial myocytes.

PR INTERVAL

The wave of depolarization, phase 0, moves through the atria, atrioventricular node, and bundle of His and the rest of the conduction system during the PR interval (Figure 7.1). It is measured from the beginning of the P wave to the beginning of ventricular depolarization. Since it contains a wave, the P wave, it is called an interval. Most of the PR interval is taken up by slow conduction through the atrioventricular node.

The segment from the end of the P wave to the onset of the QRS, the PQ segment is flat (Figure 7.1). Is there any myocardial electrical activity during the PQ segment and, if yes, why is it flat? Phase 0 is sequentially occurring in the cells of the AV node and the conduction system, during the PQ segment, but the amount of tissue is too small to generate a large enough electrical signal to be detected on the body surface, hence the flat PQ segment.

QRS

The QRS complex is the body surface recording of the sequential depolarization (phase 0) of ventricular myocytes (Figure 7.1). If there is a negative deflection at the beginning of the inscription of the ventricular complex it is called a Q wave. Any positive deflection is called an R wave—if there is a second positive deflection it is called R'. If there is a negative deflection after an R it is called an S wave. There is no such thing as a positive Q or S nor is there such a thing as a negative R wave.

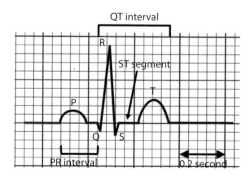

Figure 7.1 ECG waves, intervals, and segments. On the horizontal axis each small division is 1 mm and is equal to 0.04 second; 0.2 second is contained between pairs of heavy lines. Each millimeter on the vertical axis is equal to 0.1 mV. PQRST, intervals and segments are discussed in the text.

ST SEGMENT

This is a quiescent period from the end of the QRS complex to the beginning of the T wave (Figure 7.1). The ventricular cells all are in phase 2 of the action potential during the ST segment.

T WAVE

The T wave (Figure 7.1) is related to sequential development of phase 3 repolarization in ventricular myocytes. A wave due to repolarization of the atria is usually obscured by the initial portion of the QRS.

QT INTERVAL

The QT interval is measured from the beginning of the QRS complex to the end of the T wave (Figure 7.1).

STANDARD LEAD SYSTEM

A clinically effective assessment of electrical activity in the heart can be obtained with 12 views of the electrical activity, obtained with 12 different skin electrode sampling configurations or leads. An adhesive electrode containing conductive paste is applied to a previously cleaned area of the skin on each of the four limbs and at designated locations on the precordium to record the 12 leads of a standard ECG.

The appearance of the P and T waves and the QRS complex differs from lead to lead. Each lead provides a unique view of the electrical activity of the heart. **This is a topic that will be taken up after all the leads are introduced below and is also addressed in the self-study module The Mean Electrical Axis: A Story of Vectors**.

The 12 standard ECG leads are divided into 6 leads that record electrical activity reflected into the frontal plane of the torso and 6 leads that record electrical activity reflected into the horizontal plane (Figure 7.2). "Reflected into" and "plane" sound like geometry and it does take some very simple (extremely simple!) geometry to understand the clinical ECG.

The heart chambers are three-dimensional structures. For instance, as phase 0 moves from myocyte to myocyte in the atria, starting from the SA node, as phase 0 moves leftward toward the left atrium, downward toward the AV node, and rightward toward the right wall of the right atrium. That is not, however, a complete description. The action potentials also are simultaneously traversing the anterior and posterior walls of both atria. The ECG is a two-dimensional recording of the three-dimensional movement of action potentials. That is why the frontal plane leads record only that portion of the three-dimensional movement of action potentials that is reflected into (projected onto) the frontal plane.

Multiple leads are recorded in a standard ECG to obtain meaningful two-dimensional electrical views of the sequence of three-dimensional electrical events in the heart.

FRONTAL PLANE LEADS: LIMB LEADS

Picture a plane through the center of the body with the flat surfaces toward the front and rear of the body (Figure 7.2). The frontal plane leads record electrical activity reflected into that plane. The six frontal plane leads consist of three bipolar leads and three augmented unipolar leads.

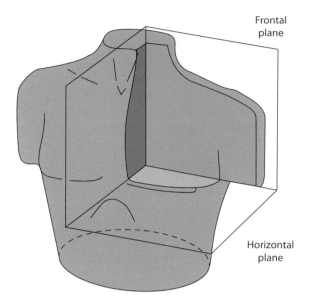

Figure 7.2 Frontal and horizontal planes. (From Malmivuo J, Plonsey R. *Bioelectromagnetism Principles and Applications of Bioelectric and Biomagnetic Fields*. 1995. by permission of Oxford University Press.)

THREE BIPOLAR LIMB LEADS I, II, AND III

Einthoven developed the bipolar limb leads. He arranged the electrodes for each lead so there was a predominantly upright QRS. This sounds arbitrary and it is, but it works because everyone since has used the same lead system (Figure 7.3). The right arm is not inherently negative and the left positive for lead I. Lead I is recorded by connecting the right arm to the negative pole of the ECG machine and the left arm to the positive pole (Figure 7.3). The left leg is connected to the positive pole of the ECG machine for leads II and III, but for lead II the right arm is connected to the negative pole and for lead III the left arm is connected to the negative pole. Note that the axes for leads I, II, and III all are at 60° to each other and form an equilateral

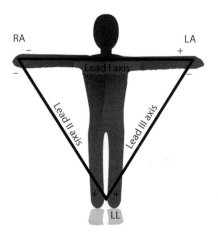

Figure 7.3 Bipolar (Einthoven) limb leads and their axes.

triangle, called Einthoven's triangle (Figure 7.3). An axis is the straight line segment connecting the electrode from one limb to another (Figure 7.3). For instance, the lead I axis is the straight line segment from the right arm electrode to the left arm electrode (Figure 7.3).

THREE AUGMENTED UNIPOLAR LIMB LEADS aVR, aVL, AND aVF

An augmented unipolar limb lead is recorded with one limb connected to the positive electrical pole of the ECG machine. The connection to the negative pole of the ECG machine is created by connecting two other limbs through resistors. Connecting two limbs together in this way creates leads whose axes bisect each of the 60° angles in Einthoven's triangle. The resistors act to increase or augment the amplitude of the recording from the one limb, hence the term "augmented." The value of the resistors was chosen through experimentation to result in ECG wave amplitudes in these leads that can be analyzed with the bipolar, Einthoven leads. The lead configurations and axes for leads aVR (Figure 7.4), aVL (Figure 7.5), and aVF (Figure 7.6) are illustrated.

Lead selection and the resistors all are part of the controls and circuitry of an ECG machine.

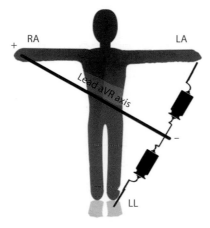

Figure 7.4 Lead aVR lead and axis.

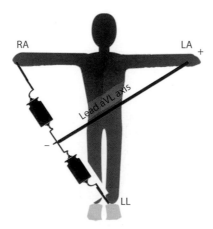

Figure 7.5 Lead aVL lead and axis.

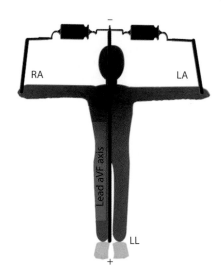

Figure 7.6 Lead aVF lead and axis.

HORIZONTAL PLANE LEADS: PRECORDIAL LEADS

The horizontal plane is perpendicular to the frontal plane and passes through the body at the approximate level of the heart (Figure 7.2). The precordial leads also are unipolar leads. The object of unipolar leads is to record voltage at different points on the body with respect to an approximation of electrical ground or zero. Electrical ground should not be affected by other electrical activity in the body, for instance, that of skeletal muscle. A true electrical ground could be obtained by connecting a wire from the patient to a ground, such as a cold-water pipe, but this creates the danger of electrocution if the ECG machine malfunctions. Consequently, no point on the body is truly at electrical ground level, but connecting the right arm, left arm, and left leg to a common point or central terminal (Figure 7.7) forms an equivalent or "body" ground or zero reference level. The point of having a central terminal is that it is little affected by electrical activity other than that of the heart and approximates a stable, zero reference level. The central terminal lead is connected to the negative pole of the ECG machine (Figure 7.7).

An exploring electrode is placed in contact with the skin at defined anatomical points on the front of the chest (Figure 7.7). The exploring electrode is connected to the positive pole of the ECG machine (Figure 7.7). The image in the upper right of Figure 7.7 is a cross-section of the chest and one is looking downward at the horizontal cut section with posterior, the spine, at the top. The exploring electrode attached to the electrode pasted on the skin of the precordium is the positive end of each precordial lead. The negative end of each precordial lead is the central terminal described above and is in the center of the thorax in the horizontal plane. The voltage difference between the central terminal and the exploring electrode is recorded for each precordial lead.

There are six precordial leads, V_1 through V_6. The precordial leads record the heart's electrical activity reflected in a horizontal plane through the heart (Figures 7.2 and 7.7). A drawing of a typical recording from V1 and V6 is illustrated (Figure 7.7). The P waves are not included.

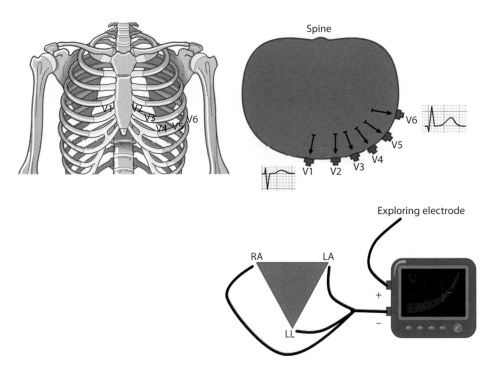

Figure 7.7 Precordial leads. The connection of the limbs to the negative terminal of the ECG machine is the central terminal described in the text. The exploring electrode is replaced by six wires in a modern ECG machine. Each wire is labeled, V1, V2, and so on, and are each connected to the respective chest electrodes. The ECG machine then records tracings from each of the six precordial leads.

MONITORING LEADS

It is common to use modified bipolar chest leads to monitor cardiac rhythm in hospitalized patients. A commonly used electrode configuration is a negative electrode near the right shoulder, a positive electrode in the V5 position, and a third reference electrode near the left shoulder. Which of the standard leads does this arrangement approximate?*

FRONTAL PLANE VECTORS

Think outside of the myocyte sarcolemma, not inside! An ECG recording is only influenced by electrical events on the outside of myocytes. In a resting myocyte, during phase 4, the outside of the myocyte is positive. K^+ has moved out through K1 channels and there is a surplus of positive ions outside of the sarcolemma (Figure 7.8). Na^+ moves in during depolarization (Figure 7.8) and at the peak of phase 0 the outside of the cell is negative because of positive charges moving into the cell (Figure 7.8).

The waves recorded in an ECG are not the result of only positive or only negative extracellular charges. The ECG waves are the result of there being an electrical potential

---

* Lead II.

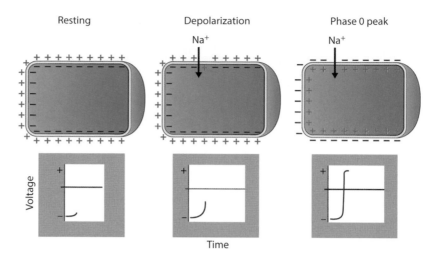

Figure 7.8 External aspect of depolarization of an atrial or ventricular myocyte in the upper images. The resting myocyte has a surplus of external K^+ and is positive outside. With depolarization Na^+ moves in and the outside develops a negative charge as the inside makes the transition from negative to positive. Internal voltage changes shown in the bottom graphs. At the peak of phase 0 there is a surplus of negative as compared with positive charges externally.

difference from one part of the atria or ventricles to another. For instance, a P wave is recorded when part of the atria is negative and part positive. Before atrial depolarization, when the outside of all the atrial cells are positive, no wave is recorded. Confusing? Think of a battery—connect something to only the positive pole and nothing happens, but then connect a bulb to the negative and positive pole—current flows through the bulb, a voltage level is created, and the bulb lights. The bulb lighting is analogous to an ECG wave recording. **This is presented with animation in the self-study module The Mean Electrical Axis: A Story of Vectors.**

The SA node normally is the first place where the outside of myocytes becomes negative as Ca^{2+} moves inward. There is too little tissue and too small an electrical signal generated by the SA node to generate a wave in the ECG recording. Then depolarization (phase 0) spreads sequentially throughout the atria. The myocytes in the portion of the atria that is depolarized are negative outside and the myocytes in the portion that is not yet depolarized are positive outside (Figure 7.9). Note that the lower and leftward portions of the atria are not yet depolarized in a "freeze frame" of an instant during atrial depolarization (Figure 7.9).

Since part of the atria is negative and part is positive, the atria behave electrically as a dipole. There is an upper, rightward, depolarized, negative pole and a lower, leftward, not-yet-depolarized, positive pole. Each small black arrow is a vector, the head of which is positive and the tail is negative (Figure 7.9).

The large white arrow is the mean vector that results if all the individual vectors are factored together (Figure 7.9). Its direction represents the average direction of the wave of depolarization at this moment and the length represents the magnitude of the electrical field associated with the dipole at this moment. This mean vector becomes a useful tool for relating what is going on electrically on the surface of the myocytes with the ECG body surface recording. **This is explained below and is illustrated with examples of vector analysis in the self-study module The Mean Electrical Axis: A Story of Vectors.**

Important: The head of the vector always points toward the positive part of the myocardium and the tail is always at the negative part. Repolarization and the T wave will be discussed later

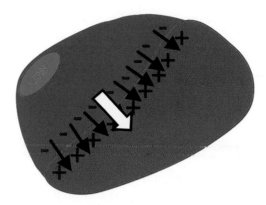

Figure 7.9 Vectors during atrial depolarization. SAN is the sinoatrial node. The large white arrow is the mean vector. Other features are discussed in the text and in the self-study module The Mean Electrical Axis: A Story of Vectors.

and the same is true—the vector points toward the positive part of the ventricular myocardium whether during depolarization or repolarization.

As noted above, the frontal plane bisects the body and is parallel to the front and back of the chest (Figure 7.2). The frontal leads record the portion of electrical activity that is reflected onto the frontal plane.

An electrical dipole has similarities to a magnetic dipole. A magnet has magnetic lines of force surrounding it. Likewise, an electrical dipole has electrical lines of force around it with current flowing from the negative portions of, for instance, atrial myocardium to the positive portions (Figure 7.9). The body tissues are excellent conductors and the electrical lines of force penetrate the tissues surrounding the heart all the way to the skin. The ECG records the resulting small electrical potential differences on the surface of the body.

The mean vector (Figure 7.9) is an understandable way to represent the magnitude and direction of an instantaneous electrical force in the heart. But the vector does not remain static. It changes amplitude and direction as depolarization progresses from myocyte to myocyte. For instance, in the atria there is no vector in between heartbeats; all the myocytes are positive outside. SA node depolarization occurs followed by depolarization of adjacent atrial myocytes. Now there are a few atrial myocytes that are negative outside and all the rest positive, and a small vector is present. Once half the atrial myocytes are depolarized and negative outside and the rest are positive outside, the vector will have grown to its maximal amplitude. Beyond the half-way point (Figure 7.9) the magnitude of the vector decreases. When all the atrial myocytes are depolarized and negative outside, the vector disappears. If that sequence of vector amplitude changes over time is projected onto a lead, the result is a P wave. The evolution of the mean vector for atrial depolarization is easier to portray than for the ventricles because the direction of the atrial mean vector does not change much.

What is meant by "projected" is discussed below. In summary, the amplitude and direction, positive or negative, of each of the ECG waves reflects the moment-by-moment evolution of the amplitude and direction of the mean vector for atrial and then ventricular depolarization and ventricular repolarization. **Projections of a mean vector onto ECG leads is a major theme of the self-study module The Mean Electrical Axis: A Story of Vectors**.

A reverse analysis also works. The mean vector at each moment during a heartbeat can be constructed from the waves recorded in an ECG.

A review of lead orientation and polarity will be helpful here.

Each ECG lead axis is oriented in a specific direction and samples skin potentials from that orientation. The orientation of the axes for leads I, II, and III are as follows:

- The axis of lead I is from shoulder to shoulder (Figure 7.3). As described above, a person's right arm (RA) is connected to the negative pole of the ECG machine and the left arm (LA) is connected to the positive pole for Lead I.
- For lead II it is RA negative, left leg (LL) positive, and the lead II axis is at 60° to lead I (Figure 7.3).
- And in lead III, the LA is negative and LL positive and the lead III axis is 60° to the axes for leads I and II (Figure 7.3).

These three bipolar leads sense electrical activity in one plane, the frontal plane of the body, and, as mentioned above, form an equilateral triangle called Einthoven's triangle (Figure 7.3). Each angle in the triangle is 60°.

As noted above, when one-half the mass of atrial myocardium is depolarized, the mean vector is the largest in magnitude, the mean vector is the longest it will be, and the peak of the P wave is recorded (Figure 7.10). The arrow representing the mean vector can be moved into the approximate center of Einthoven's triangle. The orientation and length of the vector must not change when moved (Figure 7.10). The broken lines drawn from the head and tail of the mean vector must be perpendicular to the axes they intersect (Figure 7.10). These perpendiculars project the mean vector onto each axis and the projections are represented by arrows (Figure 7.10). When the head of the projection points toward the positive end of the lead, the ECG wave is recorded as positive in that lead. In this example, the projection onto all three leads points toward the positive end of each lead. The P wave is then positive in each of the three leads (Figure 7.11). Also note that the P wave amplitude is greatest in lead II, smallest in lead III, and intermediate in lead I (Figure 7.10).

As noted above, once the atria are completely depolarized (not pictured here), with all the myocytes negative outside, there is no electrical potential difference, no vector, and the end of the P wave will be at the baseline.

The ECG signal remains at the baseline as the wave of depolarization moves slowly through the AV node (Figures 7.1, 7.2, and 7.1). The amount of AV node tissue is too small for its depolarization to be manifest on the surface of the body. In other words, the magnitude of the vector for this electrical activity is too small to influence the skin surface recording. There is rapid

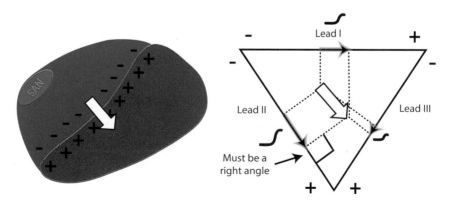

Figure 7.10 Mean vector for atrial depolarization and Einthoven's triangle. The broken lines from the head and tail of the vector must be perpendicular to each axis for a valid projection of the vector onto each lead axis.

conduction through the bundle of His, the bundle branches, and the Purkinje fibers, but, again, the amount of tissue is small and no detectable voltage change is recorded on the surface of the body. The ECG signal is flat, the PQ segment, from the end of the P wave to the beginning of the ventricular complex (Figure 7.1).

Important: The delay through the AV node ensures that ventricular contraction occurs only after atrial contraction is complete. As noted earlier, there is then time for atrial contraction to push a small amount of blood into the relaxed ventricles to finish ventricular filling. As discussed earlier, slow conduction through the AV node is due primarily to a small phase 0 slope and amplitude and small diameter cells. Also, there are relatively few gap junctions among AV node cells.

After AV node depolarization, the wave of depolarization traverses the His bundle, the bundle branches, and the Purkinje fibers. Normally the first portion of the ventricular myocardium to be depolarized is the left side of the interventricular septum. This is because the left bundle branch divides and arborizes early. Thus, depolarized myocytes on the left side of the interventricular septum are negative outside while those on the right side are still positive. The mean vector then is oriented from left to right (Figure 7.11).

The mean vector during septal depolarization, projected onto leads I and II, points to the negative end of each of those leads. This results in an initial negative deflection in these leads, a Q wave. The initial deflection is positive in lead III because the projection of the vector onto the lead III axis points toward the positive end. Thus, there will not be a Q wave in lead III and instead there is the beginning of an R wave.

Consider the remainder of the selected instants during ventricular depolarization. Following septal depolarization, depolarization moves toward the ventricular apex and then advances from the inner, subendocardial ventricular myocytes to the subepicardial, and at the same time from the apex to the base of the ventricles (Figure 7.1). Depolarization of the thinner right ventricle and the apical portions of the left ventricle occur before the remainder of the left ventricle. Myocytes in those areas are negative outside while those in the remainder of the thick left ventricle are positive and the mean vector for ventricular depolarization rotates to point leftward and downward (Figure 7.12). You should be able to reason from Figure 7.12 that there will be tall, positive deflections in leads I and II and a likely S wave in lead III. **The self-study module The Mean Electrical Axis: A Story of Vectors assists you to work through such an analysis**. The direction of the mean vector when half the ventricular myocytes are depolarized is the mean electrical axis, discussed below.

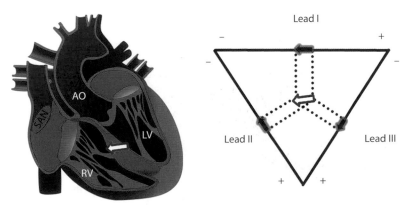

Figure 7.11 Mean vector for ventricular septal depolarization. As noted in the text, when the projection onto a lead points toward the negative end of that lead, a negative deflection is noted in the ECG. In this case the negative deflection is a Q wave in leads I and II.

(a) (b)

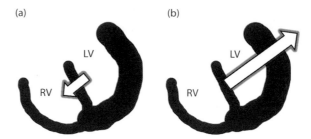

Figure 7.14 Early and late ventricular depolarization in the horizontal plane. This is a transverse section of the ventricles with the right ventricle (RV) rightward and anterior and the left ventricle (LV) leftward and posterior. The arrow in **(a)** represents the mean vector during interventricular septal depolarization and in **(b)** the arrow is the mean vector later in ventricular depolarization.

positive deflection of the QRS complex, a small R wave, in V1 (Figure 7.13). The R wave is small because the amount of tissue involved—just a portion of the interventricular septum—is small. This initial wave of depolarization is moving anteriorly and away from lead V_6 (Figures 7.13 and 7.14). Thus, there is an initial, small negative deflection of the QRS complex, a Q wave, in V_6 (Figure 7.13).

After initial depolarization of the septum, the wave of depolarization begins to spread throughout the ventricles, subendocardium to subepicardium. The mass of the left ventricle is much larger than that of the right ventricle and is leftward and posterior. The larger mass of the left ventricle takes longer for depolarization to be completed so there are not yet depolarized myocytes, positive outside, in the left ventricular free wall toward the rear. Thus, the later larger mean vector points leftward and posterior (Figure 7.14), away from V_1. This results in the large S wave in V_1 and large R wave in V_6 (Figure 7.13). The S wave in V_1 and the R wave in V_6 are large because of the large amount of tissue involved. The other precordial leads, V_2 to V_5, have intermediate patterns.

ECG PATTERNS OF NORMAL AND ABNORMAL HEART CONDUCTION

NORMAL CONDUCTION WITH NORMAL SINUS RHYTHM

When the cardiac rhythm is normal each P wave is followed at normal intervals by a ventricular complex and a T wave (Figure 7.15). Also, the rate is not abnormally slow or fast, greater than 60

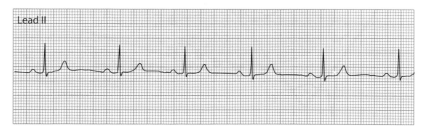

Figure 7.15 Normal conduction and normal sinus rhythm. (Reprinted from *Differential Diagnosis of Arrhythmia*, 2nd ed., Davis D, Copyright 1997, with permission from Elsevier.)

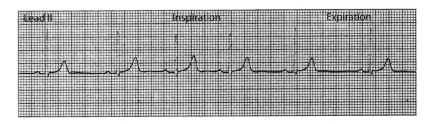

Figure 7.16 Respiratory sinus arrhythmia. (Reprinted from *Quick and Accurate 12-Lead ECG Interpretation*, 4th ed., Davis D, Copyright 2005, with permission from Elsevier.)

and less than 100 beats/minute. Less than 60 beats/minute is called bradycardia and greater than 100 beats/min is tachycardia. Since each beat of a normal rhythm starts with depolarization of the sinoatrial node, the term used is "normal sinus rhythm."

Heart rate varies from moment to moment in normal people. This normal variation in heart rate is often linked to nerve action potentials from the lungs to the brain. There are stretch receptors in the lungs with afferent nerves to cardiovascular control centers in the brain. With inspiration and stretch of lung tissue, action potentials to the brain increase. Also, brainstem neurons that control inspiration inhibit cardiac vagal neurons in the medulla. The result is less parasympathetic outflow from the central nervous system to the sinoatrial node and an increase in heart rate with inspiration (Figure 7.16). The heart rate decreases during expiration. This normal variation in heart rate is called respiratory sinus arrhythmia (Figure 7.16). There are other sinus arrhythmias not discussed here.

Labelling this respiratory sinus arrhythmia is unfortunate since it is normal. It is more pronounced in normal infants and in adults with slow resting heart rates, such as endurance-trained people. In fact, recent studies indicate that heart rate variation tends to disappear in heart disease. Heart failure is accompanied by reduced resting heart rate variation for reasons that have yet to be determined.

ATRIOVENTRICULAR AND INTRAVENTRICULAR CONDUCTION BLOCKS

Physiological changes, drugs, and disease can adversely affect the AV node or conduction system. The result may be varying degrees of impairment of transmission of action potentials from the atria to the ventricles. Such impairment is called heart block and some of the more common degrees and types of heart block are illustrated.

FIRST DEGREE ATRIOVENTRICULAR BLOCK

There is prolonged conduction from the atria to the ventricles in first degree heart block (Figure 7.17). The P wave at the arrow starts on a heavy vertical line and the tiny Q wave starts 5.5 divisions later, which equals a PR interval of 0.22 seconds. The PR interval lengthens as heart rate slows, but normally does not exceed 0.20 sec. Some drugs and inflammation, such as in acute rheumatic fever, will slow conduction through the atrioventricular node. The lengthening with heart rate slowing is related to less sympathetic and more parasympathetic input to the AV node. Both less catecholamine interaction with AV node beta receptors and more acetylcholine effects on the AV node result in a reduction in I_{L-Ca} and a decrease in the upslope and amplitude of phase 0. Thus, AV node conduction velocity is reduced.

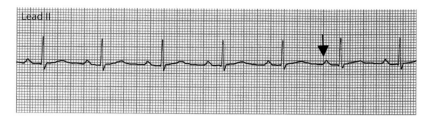

Figure 7.17 First degree atrioventricular block. The duration of the PR interval after the arrow is 0.22 seconds. (Reprinted from *Differential Diagnosis of Arrhythmias*, 2nd ed., Davis D, Copyright 1997, with permission from Elsevier.)

There is no functional impairment with first degree atrioventricular block nor is it likely to progress to a higher degree of block. Some experts are reluctant to call this a block and refer to this ECG pattern as simply a prolonged PR interval.

SECOND DEGREE ATRIOVENTRICULAR BLOCK

In first degree atrioventricular block every P wave is followed by ventricular depolarization. In second degree atrioventricular block there are instances where conduction from atria to ventricles fails to occur and a ventricular action potential does not follow a P wave. The cause varies and can be due to such things as drug toxicity, ischemia, and inflammation affecting some part of the conduction system. Second degree heart block also can be related to the effects of the autonomic nervous system on a normal atrioventricular node. There are two types of second degree atrioventricular block.

Mobitz Type I or Wenckebach atrioventricular block

This is a relatively benign form of atrioventricular block usually involving altered atrioventricular node physiology. It is likely due to the effects of increased parasympathetic nerve activity on the AV node. In this type of atrioventricular block there is a progressive increase of the PR interval until finally a beat occurs with no conduction to and no electrical activity recorded in the ventricles (Figure 7.18).

In this rhythm strip there is a small amount of upward drift of the baseline, which is a recording artifact and not due to an abnormality. The P wave at the arrow (Figure 7.18) is the beginning of a prolonged PR interval, but is followed by conduction to and depolarization of the ventricles; there is an RS complex followed by a T wave. Then the next four PR intervals become progressively longer. Finally, the fifth P wave after the P at the arrow is not followed by

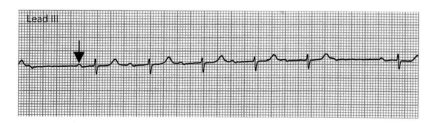

Figure 7.18 Second degree, Mobitz Type 1, Wenckebach atrioventricular block. (Reprinted from *Differential Diagnosis of Arrhythmias*, 2nd ed., Davis D, Copyright 1997, with permission from Elsevier.)

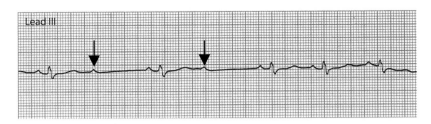

Figure 7.19 Second degree, Mobitz Type II, atrioventricular block. The arrows point to nonconducted beats described in the text. (Reprinted from *Differential Diagnosis of Arrhythmias*, 2nd ed., Davis D, Copyright 1997, with permission from Elsevier.)

a ventricular complex. There is no conduction from the atria to the ventricles and a "dropped beat" occurs. After a long pause the sequence likely begins again although the ratio of conducted to nonconducted beats can vary.

Wenckebach tends to occur at a slow heart rate when parasympathetic input to the SA node predominates. Wenckebach atrioventricular block can occur in normal young people and is often observed in infants and in endurance athletes. It can be due to conduction system pathology and lead to more serious problems in older patients.

Mobitz Type II atrioventricular block

In this form of second degree heart block there is a sudden failure of conduction from the atria to the ventricles without preceding PR interval prolongation. The P waves at the arrows in Figure 7.19 are not followed by ventricular depolarization and repolarization. The other P waves are followed by normal conduction with normal, stable PR intervals (Figure 7.19). There is no progressive elongation of the PR interval as in Wenckebach, Mobitz type I atrioventricular block.

Mobitz Type II atrioventricular block can occur as a toxic effect of drugs, ischemia, inflammation, and so on. It is likely that the disturbed conduction is related to pathophysiologic or pathologic changes in the His bundle or other parts of the conduction system rather than physiologic effects on the atrioventricular node. The presence of Mobitz type II atrioventricular block is a cause for concern because more complete block may appear—every third beat, every second beat, and so on. This can lead to complete atrioventricular block and associated complications discussed next.

COMPLETE HEART BLOCK, COMPLETE ATRIOVENTRICULAR BLOCK, OR COMPLETE ATRIOVENTRICULAR DISSOCIATION (THE MORE GENERALLY USED TERMS RATHER THAN THIRD-DEGREE HEART BLOCK)

Damage to the atrioventricular node, bundle of His, or both bundle branches can cause a complete failure of conduction from the atria to the ventricles. In Figure 7.20, arrows mark the location of atrial depolarizations occurring at about 100/minute. RST waves are occurring regularly, but at a much slower rate than the P waves, approximately 44/minute. The atria are depolarizing regularly at their own rate and the ventricles are doing the same, but at their own much slower rate without a fixed relationship to atrial depolarizations. A likely source of ventricular pacing in this situation are Purkinje fibers. The fourth arrow from the left marks the occurrence of an R wave likely superimposed on a P wave. Notice that the R wave is taller than the others. Several of the P waves are superimposed on T waves.

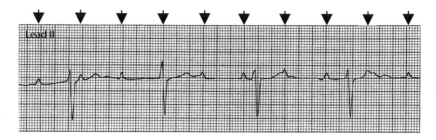

Figure 7.20 Complete atrioventricular dissociation or complete heart block. The arrows mark the occurrence of atrial depolarizations. (Reprinted from *Quick and Accurate 12-Lead ECG Interpretation*, 4th ed., Davis D, Copyright 2005, with permission from Elsevier.)

BUNDLE BRANCH BLOCKS

A conduction block in the right or left bundle branch leads to changes from normal in all the ECG leads. The changes from normal in the precordial leads are distinctive and usually used to characterize right and left bundle branch block.

Complete right bundle branch block (CRBBB)

CRBBB can occur in people who have no clinical evidence of heart disease. In these otherwise normal people, CRBBB does not predict future heart problems. CRBBB can also occur due to dysfunction of the right bundle branch related to right ventricular pressure or volume overload and hypertrophy. Ischemia involving the right bundle branch can result in CRBBB. In the presence of structural heart disease, CRBBB can progress to complete heart block if the left bundle or bundle of His also becomes involved.

In CRBBB there is a small R wave in lead V_1 and a Q wave in V_6 just as in a normal ECG (Figure 7.21a and b). The R and Q wave are unchanged from normal because the left bundle branch is functional and depolarization begins, as usual, on the left, posterior side of the interventricular septum. Again, as in a normal ECG, the R in V_1 is followed by a deep S wave due to the later depolarization of the leftward, posterior left ventricle (Figures 7.13, 7.14, and 7.21b). This movement of depolarization posteriorly also accounts for the R wave in V_6 (Figures 7.13, 7.14, and 7.21b). The left bundle branch conduction system is normal and action potentials travel rapidly to the left septal and left ventricular myocardium.

The right bundle branch is completely blocked and action potentials cannot be distributed by the right bundle rapid conduction system. The action potentials reach the right ventricle by traveling relatively slowly through the right ventricular myocardium. So right ventricular depolarization is delayed and appears as a second, wide R′ wave in V_1 and a deep, wide S wave in V_6 (Figure 7.21b). The right ventricle is an anterior structure and the late depolarization moves toward V1 and away from V6. The result is the classic configuration for CRBBB in the precordial leads: an RSR′ in V1, the mirror image in V6, and a wider than normal ventricular complex (Figure 7.21b).

Complete left bundle branch block (CLBBB)

CLBBB rarely occurs in the absence of structural heart disease. Any heart disease that results in left ventricular hypertrophy (aortic valvular disease, high blood pressure, cardiomyopathy, etc.) can result in CLBBB. Myocardial ischemia due to obstruction of a coronary artery can involve left bundle myocytes and result in CLBBB.

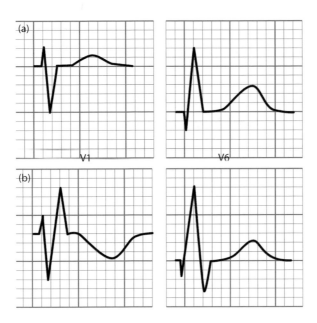

Figure 7.21 Complete right bundle branch block. **(a)** is the normal V1 and V6 and (b) is the configuration in complete right bundle branch block in V1 and V6. P waves are not shown here and would be normal. The inverted T wave in V1 in **(b)** is not characteristic of CRBBB and may not be present.

In the presence of CLBBB, initial ventricular depolarization occurs on the right, anterior side of the interventricular septum instead of the left, posterior side. Consequently, there is no R wave in V1 (Figure 7.22b). Septal activation proceeds from right, anterior to left, posterior and the vector for septal depolarization persistently points toward V6 and away from V1.

The intact right bundle branch conduction system depolarizes the right ventricle sooner than the left ventricle. This results initially in depolarized, negative tissue anteriorly and not-yet-depolarized, positive left ventricular tissue posteriorly. This negative to positive, front to back orientation results in a deep, wide QS wave in V1 (Figure 7.22b). It is wide because depolarization of the left ventricle without the left conduction system proceeds slowly among the left ventricular myocytes.

The notch in the QS wave (Figure 7.22b) is probably due to the less organized travel of depolarization through the left ventricular myocardium that can occur in the absence of the left bundle branch conduction system. A notch and any T wave changes are not always present. The configuration of ventricular depolarization in V6 is, as usual, the mirror image of that in V1 (Figure 7.22).

CLBBB can contribute to left ventricular dysfunction in heart failure. A relatively new therapy involves using an implanted power source with wires connected to left ventricular myocardium to "resynchronize" left ventricular activation by inducing a more normal sequence of ventricular action potentials.

WOLFF–PARKINSON–WHITE OR PREEXCITATION

This is an excellent example of correlation of an ECG pattern with abnormal anatomy. In Wolff–Parkinson–White (WPW) there are abnormal congenital muscle connections (bundles of Kent) from the atria to the ventricles, which bridge the annulus fibrosus. Conduction in

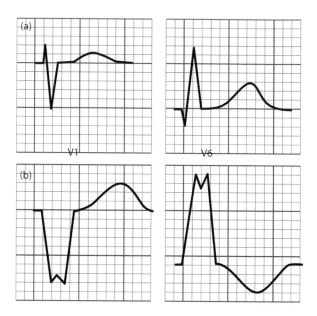

Figure 7.22 Complete left bundle branch block. **(a)** is the normal V1 and V6 and **(b)** is the configuration in complete left bundle branch block in V1 and V6. P waves are not shown here and would be normal. Any T wave changes from normal are not diagnostic.

these accessory pathways leads to earlier than normal ventricular activation or preexcitation. Conduction velocity is higher in the muscular connections than in the AV node, so ventricular depolarization begins sooner than normal in ventricular tissue and bypasses the normal conduction system.

Conduction velocity in ventricular muscle is faster than in the AV node, but is slower than in the conduction system. Thus, initial ventricular depolarization is slower than normal and generates a slurred initial portion of ventricular depolarization, the delta wave (Figure 7.23, arrow). Meanwhile, action potentials slowly travel through the AV node and then enter the conduction system just as normal. Action potentials are then rapidly distributed by the conduction system to ventricular myocardium and ventricular depolarization after the delta wave is brisk (Figure 7.23). The later portion of the ventricular complex is narrow (Figure 7.23). The delta wave plus

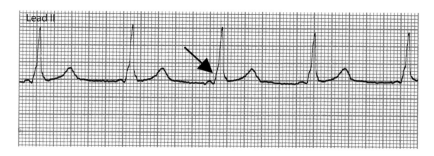

Figure 7.23 Wolff–Parkinson–White or preexcitation. The arrow points to the slurred beginning of ventricular depolarization, the delta wave, so-called because of its similarity to the first part of the Greek letter Δ. (Reprinted from *Differential Diagnosis of Arrhythmias*, 2nd ed., Davis D, Copyright 1997, with permission from Elsevier.)

the later faster inscription of ventricular depolarization result in a prolonged total QRS duration, greater than 0.11 seconds.

WPW is diagnosed from the ECG when there is: (1) a short PR interval, (2) a wide QRS, and (3) a slurred initial QRS complex (delta wave) (Figure 7.23). WPW predisposes individuals to develop tachycardia. The tachycardias can arise due to reentry, which is discussed below.

ECG PATTERNS OF ABNORMAL RHYTHMS: ARRHYTHMIAS

ATRIAL ARRHYTHMIAS

PREMATURE ATRIAL BEATS

Premature atrial beats can occur in normal hearts, but also can be secondary to the effects of drugs or disease. In a premature atrial beat the P wave occurs earlier than expected (arrows in Figure 7.24), but the premature P wave is followed by the usual waveforms of ventricular depolarization and repolarization.

LOWER ATRIAL PREMATURE BEAT

The arrow indicates lower atrial premature beat (Figure 7.25). The interval from the preceding P wave to the inverted P wave at the arrow is shorter than the other P to P intervals (Figure 7.25). The negative polarity of the P wave in this lead II tracing suggests that it originates in the lower

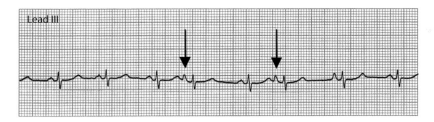

Figure 7.24 Premature atrial beats. The arrows point to the P waves occurring earlier than expected. (Reprinted from *Differential Diagnosis of Arrhythmias*, 2nd ed., Davis D, Copyright 1997, with permission from Elsevier.)

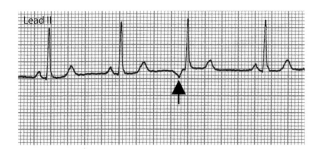

Figure 7.25 Lower Atrial Premature Beat. A lower atrial premature beat is indicated by the arrow. (Reprinted from *Differential Diagnosis of Arrhythmias*, 2nd ed., Davis D, Copyright 1997, with permission from Elsevier.)

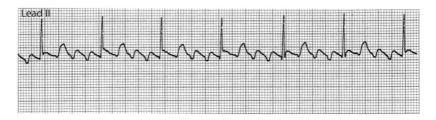

Figure 7.26 Atrial flutter. In this case there are four atrial depolarizations for each ventricular or 4:1 conduction. The atrial depolarizations are called flutter waves. One atrial flutter wave is obscured by each QRS complex. Conduction to the ventricles is not more frequent because of the long refractoriness of the atrioventricular node. (Reprinted from *Differential Diagnosis of Arrhythmias*, 2nd ed., Davis D, Copyright 1997, with permission from Elsevier.)

part of the atria because atrial depolarization is then likely from the bottom of the atria upward toward the right. That would result in a mean vector for atrial depolarization pointing toward the negative end of lead II.

ATRIAL FLUTTER

Atrial flutter typically originates in the right atrium. In atrial flutter, action potentials travel a circular, usually counterclockwise path in the right atrial myocardium affected by drug toxicity, disease, or surgical scarring. It is an example of a reentrant arrhythmia (reentry is discussed later) in that depolarizations follow a circular path and re-excite previously depolarized atrial myocytes. This repetitive circular loop results in depolarization of the atria at a rate of 220 to 350 per minute (Figure 7.26). The frequency is related to path length, a function of the size of the atrium, and conduction velocity.

The ventricular rate in the example presented here is 70/minute (Figure 7.26). The frequent atrial depolarizations create a typical "sawtooth" pattern at a frequency in this example of 280/minute (Figure 7.26). That corresponds to four atrial depolarizations for every one ventricular or 4:1 conduction. One atrial depolarization is hidden by the simultaneously occurring ventricular depolarization. Every atrial depolarization is usually not followed by a ventricular depolarization due to the long total refractoriness of the atrioventricular node. This is a great example of the atrioventricular node protecting the ventricles from beating too rapidly when there is a rapid atrial arrhythmia. Rarely 1:1 conduction occurs with an excessively rapid ventricular rate.

ATRIAL FIBRILLATION

In atrial fibrillation (Figure 7.27) there is random, chaotic atrial electrical activity. The atrioventricular node is randomly bombarded by action potentials. Some of the atrial action potentials induce atrioventricular node action potentials, which then conduct to the ventricles. Others find the atrioventricular node refractory. The resulting ventricular depolarizations are irregularly spaced (Figure 7.27). Since the atrial electrical activity is random and chaotic, there is no organized depolarization wave front in the atria and there are no P waves. Likewise, there is no effective atrial contraction, although that is not measured by the ECG, but can be measured by other means.

There usually are baseline fluctuations, called fibrillation waves, but no consistent P wave precedes each ventricular complex (Figure 7.27). Atrial fibrillation can occur, for instance, whenever there is hypertrophy or dilatation of the atria. Recognition of this arrhythmia should be relatively easy: no P waves + irregular R-R intervals = atrial fibrillation.

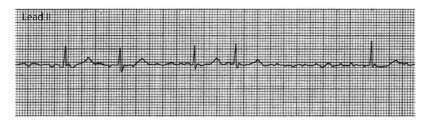

Figure 7.27 Atrial fibrillation. The baseline fluctuations are fibrillation waves reflective of the random chaotic atrial depolarizations. (Reprinted from *Quick and Accurate 12-Lead ECG Interpretation*, 4th ed., Davis D, Copyright 2005, with permission from Elsevier.)

The chaotic atrial electrical activity occurs with a usual frequency of 400 to 600 per minute. The fact that the ventricular rate does not follow at that high frequency is another example of how the long total refractoriness of the atrioventricular node is protective.

ABNORMAL VENTRICULAR BEATS

VENTRICULAR PREMATURE BEATS

A ventricular premature beat (Figure 7.28), as the name indicates, is a ventricular beat that occurs earlier than expected. There is no preceding P wave because the premature ventricular beat most often originates within a ventricular muscle focus. Note that the wave preceding each of the two premature ventricular beats (arrows in Figure 7.28) is a T wave related to the previous sinus beat, not a P wave. A ventricular premature beat originating from a ventricular muscle focus looks very different (arrows in Figure 7.28) than a normal QRS complex. Its shape and long duration are related to the slower moving, less organized wave front of ventricular depolarization when the conduction system is not distributing the action potentials. A ventricular premature beat originating in the conduction system would look very much like the other, normal ventricular depolarizations, but would be premature and without a preceding P wave.

Occasional, isolated ventricular premature beats can occur normally. They are of concern when they occur in the presence of heart disease or potentially cardiotoxic drugs.

VENTRICULAR TACHYCARDIA

Three or more ventricular premature beats in succession constitute ventricular tachycardia. In ventricular tachycardia (Figure 7.29), there is an abnormal pacemaker somewhere in the ventricular myocardium. Usually, the abnormal pacemaker is an area of damaged and unstable ventricular muscle. There is no P wave preceding each R wave (Figure 7.29) since the ventricular

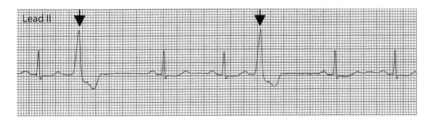

Figure 7.28 Premature ventricular beats indicated by the arrows. (Reprinted from *Differential Diagnosis of Arrhythmias*, 2nd ed., Davis D, Copyright 1997, with permission from Elsevier.)

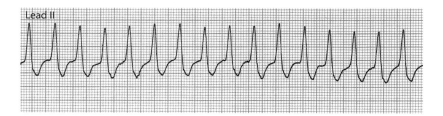

Figure 7.29 Ventricular tachycardia. (Reprinted from *Differential Diagnosis of Arrhythmias*, 2nd ed., Davis D, Copyright 1997, with permission from Elsevier.)

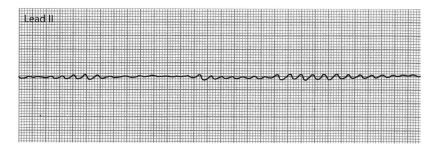

Figure 7.30 Ventricular fibrillation. (Reprinted from *Differential Diagnosis of Arrhythmias*, 2nd ed., Davis D, Copyright 1997, with permission from Elsevier.)

depolarizations are arising from ventricular muscle. The atria are depolarizing but the P waves are mostly obscured by the ventricular waveforms. The ventricular rate may be high enough to limit the time for ventricular filling, but compromised ventricular filling would have to be evaluated with other than the ECG. Reduced ventricular filling can result in inadequate ventricular pumping, particularly if there is associated ventricular muscle dysfunction, and circulatory collapse with shock may occur. If arterial blood pressure falls significantly with ventricular tachycardia, perfusion of the coronary vasculature will fall and ventricular tachycardia then can deteriorate into ventricular fibrillation and death.

VENTRICULAR FIBRILLATION

In ventricular fibrillation (Figure 7.30), ventricular electrical activity is random and chaotic. There is no organized, sequential wave of depolarization.

There is no direct information from the ECG about function, but there is no effective organized ventricular contraction and no effective pumping of blood by the heart in ventricular fibrillation. Obviously, ventricular fibrillation results in death within minutes. Fibrillation waves, giving the appearance of an undulating baseline (Figure 7.30), can be fine or coarse, just as in atrial fibrillation.

MECHANISMS OF ARRHYTHMIAS

REENTRY

Most arrhythmias occur due to reentry. One example of reentry involves the junction of Purkinje fibers with ventricular myocardium. Purkinje myocytes are highly branched. Consider

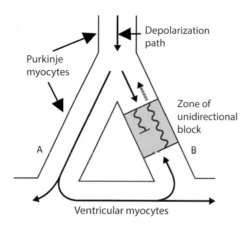

Figure 7.31 Model of unidirectional block in a branched Purkinje fiber. In the zone of unidirectional block (shaded) the zigzag lines indicate the variable or blocked conduction that can occur. The arrow exiting at the top of the zone of unidirectional block is shaded to indicate a depolarization emerging from the zone, which may or may not induce depolarizations in the normal Purkinje myocytes.

a simple model of a region where a Purkinje myocyte branches and joins ventricular muscle (Figure 7.31). Distal Purkinje branches are susceptible to one-way block, called unidirectional block (Figure 7.31). This can develop in an area injured, for instance, by hypoxia secondary to inadequate coronary blood flow.

Depolarizations traverse the Purkinje branches (Figure 7.31) and branch A merges with normal ventricular myocytes. Depolarization is blocked at the zone of unidirectional block in branch B (Figure 7.31). Depolarizations can propagate in any path that has myocytes ready to develop an action potential, since all myocytes are interconnected by gap junctions. Hence action potentials propagate retrograde in the distal part of branch B (Figure 7.31).

One mechanism for a zone of unidirectional block is that hypoxia can affect the excitability and refractoriness of myocytes and the effects of hypoxia can vary among myocytes. The variably damaged cells in the zone of unidirectional block (Figure 7.31) are temporarily not capable of being depolarized by the depolarizations moving down branch B (Figure 7.31). The depolarizations in branch A (Figure 7.31) traverse a long pathway in interconnected normal Purkinje and ventricular myocytes and eventually propagate retrograde in the distal portion of branch B (Figure 7.31). The Purkinje myocytes in the distal portion of branch B, past the area of unidirectional block, are normal, interconnected by gap junctions, have not yet depolarized, and are not refractory.

Enough time may have passed so that the damaged myocytes in the zone of unidirectional block have recovered enough so that depolarizations arriving retrograde (Figure 7.31) can induce action potentials in the unidirectional block zone. The action potentials induced in the damaged cells in the unidirectional block zone are not normal and can vary among myocytes, so conduction through the blocked zone is usually slower than normal and varies among the damaged myocytes (Figure 7.31, wavy line).

Depolarizations that get through the zone of unidirectional block now reenter the proximal part of branch B (Figure 7.31, shaded arrow). The long circular path and slow retrograde conduction of the action potential through the unidirectional block area can take enough time for the normal Purkinje cells to reach the end of the relative refractory period. The retrograde conduction into the proximal part of branch B (Figure 7.31, shaded arrow) may now produce depolarizations that again conduct down the normal branch A and begin the cycle again.

Each cycle is transmitted to all other ventricular myocytes through gap junctions and a premature ventricular beat is generated with each "circle."

This circular or circus movement can produce, for example, one or more ventricular premature beats or, if sustained, ventricular tachycardia. Gap junctions facilitate the transmission of each circular depolarization to all other ventricular cells.

Circus movement also can occur in the absence of an area of unidirectional block. All that is needed is an area of abnormal cells with variable excitability and refractoriness. As depolarizations make their way in a tortuous, abnormally long pathway among and around these abnormal cells they may find a previously depolarized, but now vulnerable area that can be reexcited. Reentry can occur in other than Purkinje myocytes. It can occur in ventricular and atrial myocardium, in conduction tissue, and in nodal tissue. Atrial flutter was discussed earlier and is an arrhythmia involving reentrant, circus movement of depolarization, usually in the right atrium.

Reentry or circus movement is prone to occur in the presence of:

- An abnormally long conduction pathway,
- Decreased conduction velocity, and
- A short absolute refractory period of the normal myocardium.

Locally blocked or abnormally slow conduction can occur in numerous abnormal circumstances. For instance, in the presence of coronary artery obstruction there is a lack of supply of oxygenated blood to a region of the myocardium. Abnormal function in the myocytes in such a region may result in a zone of unidirectional block or create conditions for an abnormal, long, tortuous, slow conduction pathway and reentry can result. Inflammatory injury can produce similar effects.

Some drugs used to treat arrhythmias are designed to prolong the absolute refractory period to prevent reentry phenomena. If the treatment works, depolarizations will either find myocytes still refractory at the area of unidirectional block or depolarizations exiting a zone of unidirectional block (Figure 7.31, shaded arrow) will find the normal cells still refractory. Also, the abnormal conduction pathway can be shortened by maneuvers that increase myocardial oxygenation, such as opening a blocked coronary artery. Clinical cardiac electrophysiologists can catheterize a patient, insert catheters with contact electrodes, record electrograms from the inner surface of a heart chamber, map electrical activity, and locate circus patterns. They then can use catheters that emit high frequency energy to damage minute amounts of myocardium in the reentry path and stop the circus movement of depolarization.

TRIGGERED ACTIVITY

Triggered activity refers to a second action potential that occurs during phase 2, 3, or 4 (Figure 7.32). Something abnormal happens during a myocardial action potential that "triggers" a second action potential to occur during or immediately after that same action potential.

Triggered activity falls into two broad categories, early and delayed afterdepolarizations (Figure 7.32). Early triggered ventricular or atrial action potentials occur during phase 2 or 3 (Figure 7.32) at a time when the cell should be refractory. A delayed triggered action potential occurs early in phase 4, closely following the preceding action potential (Figure 7.32).

Myoplasmic Ca^{2+} overload is a feature common to both early and delayed afterdepolarizations. Ca^{2+} influx during an action potential is an essential step in normal excitation-contraction-coupling. The Ca^{2+} entering, mostly during phase 2, induces the release of Ca^{2+} from sarcoplasmic reticulum terminal cisternae and this Ca^{2+}-induced-Ca^{2+}-release leads to myocyte contraction. But too much cytoplasmic Ca^{2+} can be a problem.

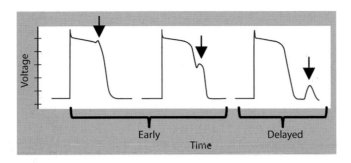

Figure 7.32 Triggered activity. Early and delayed afterdepolarizations are indicated.

Excessive cytoplasmic Ca^{2+} results in more than normal Na^+ exchange with Ca^{2+} across the sarcolemma. As noted earlier, this exchange involves 3 Na^+ entering for 1 Ca^{2+} exiting and is depolarizing. Also, excessive levels of cytoplasmic Ca^{2+} can induce a transient inward movement of Na^+, the mechanism for which is not well defined. Increased cytoplasmic Ca^{2+} normally stimulates the sarcoplasmic reticulum to take up Ca^{2+}, which is a normal mechanism for relaxation. In the presence of excessive cytoplasmic Ca^{2+}, the sarcoplasmic reticulum becomes overloaded with Ca^{2+} and the terminal cisternae begin to spontaneously release Ca^{2+} into the cytoplasm, creating repetitive cycles of Ca^{2+} release and uptake. Release of Ca^{2+} into the cytoplasm leads to more 3 Na^+/1 Ca^{2+} exchange as noted above.

Cytoplasmic Ca^{2+} overload can occur, for example, as a complication of drugs such as digoxin or in the presence of increased sympathetic activity. Ischemia and hypoxia can change myocyte metabolism in such a way as to lead to Ca^{2+} overload.

EARLY AFTERDEPOLARIZATIONS

Early afterdepolarizations (Figure 7.32) tend to occur with action potential prolongation. A decrease in heart rate normally is accompanied by prolongation of atrial and ventricular myocyte action potentials, particularly phase 2. Normal prolongation of phase 2 with a low heart rate derives from effects related to I_K.

Phase 2 may be excessively prolonged as heart rate slows. This excessive prolongation can occur, for instance, due to certain drugs (some antiarrhythmics, antibiotics, antihistamines, etc.). Some myocardial tissues are more prone to this such as left ventricular mid-ventricular myocytes, the M fibers, that normally have longer action potentials than the subepicardial and subendocardial ventricular fibers.

As noted earlier, L-type Ca^{2+} channels begin opening during phase 0 of the ventricular action potential and they deactivate toward the end of phase 2. Abnormal prolongation of phase 2 can reactivate L-type Ca^{2+} channels and produce a depolarizing Ca^{2+} current and an early afterdepolarization. The fast Na^+ channels are inactivated during phase 2, but an early afterdepolarization can progress to a Ca^{2+} action potential. Once atrial or ventricular myocytes enter phase 3 and the transmembrane potential reaches -60 to -70 mV, some fast Na^+ channels reactivate and can depolarize and produce a phase 3 early afterdepolarization. If the phase 3 afterdepolarization is large enough, an Na^+ action potential can result.

One treatment strategy consists of the insertion of a pacing catheter to increase heart rate. Phase 2 shortens as heart rate increases. This type of temporary treatment would be appropriate for a hospitalized patient.

DELAYED AFTERDEPOLARIZATIONS

Delayed afterdepolarizations are also induced by high intracellular Ca^{2+} concentrations as described above. One scenario could involve a patient with an acute myocardial infarction, with the accompanying increased sympathetic response to pain or due to autonomic reflexes. Ca^{2+} overload here is related to the fact that catecholamines increase L-type Ca^{2+} channel opening and prolong how long they are open. More Ca^{2+} enters the myocytes. Catecholamines also enhance Ca^{2+} uptake by the sarcoplasmic reticulum. The sarcoplasmic reticulum becomes overloaded with Ca^{2+} and the terminal cisternae begin spontaneously releasing Ca^{2+} into the cytoplasm. In this scenario, heart rate will be fast related to increased sympathetic effects on the sinoatrial node.

What can be confusing in a patient with bradycardia is that the prolonged time for Ca^{2+} entry into myocytes and the resulting cytoplasmic Ca^{2+} overload, discussed above, may lead to delayed afterdepolarizations as well as to early afterdepolarizations. Clinical decision-making here can be perplexing! Afterdepolarizations can be treated with, for instance, drugs that partially block Ca^{2+} or Na^+ movement across the sarcolemma.

LONG QT SYNDROME

Repolarization is delayed and the plateau is abnormally prolonged in this syndrome, which can be either genetic or acquired. The triggered extra beats that occur in the long QT syndrome occur in phase 2 or 3. This is a special case of early afterdepolarizations. In the most common genetic form of this problem there is decreased K channel function and repolarization is delayed. In a less common genetic defect of fast Na^+ channels their function is enhanced such that they open during phase 2 or 3 of the action potential instead of remaining inactivated. In the acquired form of the long QT syndrome, similar channel changes are induced by effects of drugs.

A delay in repolarization results in either a long phase 2 or prolongation of phase 3. In either case the time from the onset of ventricular depolarization on the ECG to the end of the T wave is longer than normal (Figure 7.33).

The patient can develop afterdepolarizations that can progress to a multiform, multifocal ventricular tachycardia called Torsades de Pointes (Figures 7.34 and 7.35). Torsades de Pointes is a rapid polymorphic, polyphasic ventricular tachycardia. "Torsades de Pointes" refers to the varying amplitude of the ventricular complexes giving the appearance of their "twisting around a point" or imaginary baseline, as in a party streamer (Figure 7.34). The danger is that this rapid ventricular arrhythmia can limit ventricular filling time enough to decrease cardiac output and arterial pressure. Decreased coronary vascular perfusion and myocardial hypoxia then can lead to ventricular fibrillation and sudden death.

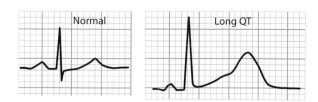

Figure 7.33 Normal and congenital long QT syndrome ECG tracings. The larger R wave in the abnormal recording is not a significant finding.

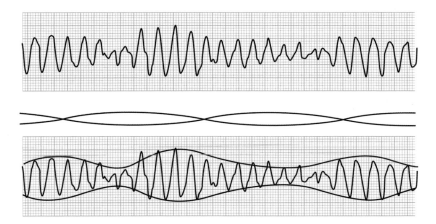

Figure 7.34 Torsade de Pointes. The top drawing illustrates the variable shape of the ventricular depolarizations (polymorphic) and the frequency (polyphasic). A twisted party streamer is depicted in the middle of the figure. The lower tracing illustrates the undulating pattern of the ECG waves that led the authors who originally reported this arrhythmia to describe it as twisting around a point, similar to a twisted paper party streamer.

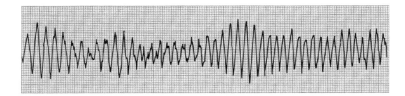

Figure 7.35 Torsades de Pointes. (From Goldberger AL. *Clinical Electrocardiography.* 7th ed. Philadelphia: Mosby Elsevier; 2006. [16–18, p. 199]).

Clinicians need to be aware of drugs that prolong myocardial action potentials, and if a drug prolongs the QT interval treatment must be carefully monitored. Identification and treatment of genetically affected individuals is important to prevent sudden death. There are age and gender differences in the manifestations of the genetic syndrome that should be taken into consideration. Clinical research continues, but treatments that are being studied include the use of β blocking drugs, left cardiac sympathetic denervation, and implantation of a cardioverter defibrillator.

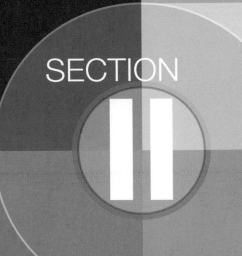

SECTION II

CARDIOVASCULAR SYSTEM

About 5 liters of blood per minute circulate around your body even when you are resting. In other words, 5 one-liter soft drink bottles full of blood moved every 60 seconds! During exercise that amount can increase to 20 liters per minute or more! Moved from where to where? At any given moment, most of the blood in your body, 60% to 70%, resides in the veins. A major function of the heart is to receive blood at low pressure from the venous compartment, transport it through the lungs, and increase the pressure as the blood is ejected into the arterial conduits. The blood then flows from the high pressure arterial side of the circulation back to the low pressure venous side, and so on, continuously in a circle, just as demonstrated first by William Harvey in the seventeenth century.

What does the above have to do with the pathophysiology of heart disease? Just this—the body's demand for nutrition supplied by blood flow continues unabated when ventricular function becomes abnormal. Overall body metabolism persists, the demand of the body for oxygen continues, and the body's feedback mechanisms strive to maintain blood flow into the microcirculation for gas and other exchange. The feedback mechanisms act mostly via the autonomic nerves to the heart, blood vessels, and adrenal gland. Quite simply, the body has no mechanisms to rest a weakening heart. There is a continuing drive to produce cardiac output adequate for body metabolism. Moreover, this drive continues in the presence of abnormal heart valves or heart muscle pathology. These continuing demands on the abnormal heart lead to ventricular dysfunction, adverse myocardial myocyte remodeling, and the symptoms we diagnose as heart disease.

As you can understand from the above, one cannot diagnose and treat heart disease without understanding how the normal circulation works, including some of the simple physics of circulating fluid, how the heart pumps blood, and the characteristics of the peripheral circulation, controls in the circulation, individual organ circulation, and the microcirculation.

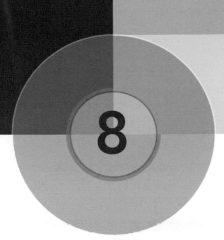

How the circulation works

BLOOD PRESSURE

A little physics is useful here. Pressure can be measured as the height of a column of fluid connected to a pressurized "container," such as a blood vessel (Figure 8.1). Use of the height of a fluid column is based on pressure = $\rho g h$; ρ is fluid density, g is acceleration due to gravity, and h is the height of the fluid column.

The density, ρ, of a fluid such as mercury or water and the acceleration due to gravity, g, are known and constant, so pressure can be expressed simply as the height (h) of a column of liquid. Two basic types of pressure measuring devices are illustrated (Figure 8.1a and b).

ENERGY

Most of the energy in the circulation ultimately derives from the hydrolysis of ATP in heart muscle and conversion of high energy phosphate bonds by sarcomeres into heart muscle work. Work is done by heart muscle on blood contained within the heart and that work is transformed into two types of energy: pressure potential energy and energy related to movement, kinetic energy. A third type of energy is not derived from heart muscle function. It is derived from the effects of gravity on blood in the circulation. Energy in the circulation will be defined first and then flow will be discussed, including a discussion of gravity's effects on the circulation.

Total fluid energy is defined as follows:

Total Energy = Pressure Potential Energy + Kinetic Energy + Gravitational Potential Energy

$$W \quad = \quad P \quad + \quad (\rho v^2)/2 \quad + \quad \rho g h$$

P, pressure potential energy, develops due to the work done on the blood in the ventricle by the contracting heart muscle myocytes during systole. Contracting ventricular muscle squeezes blood within the ventricular chambers, which cannot decrease in volume because the valves are all closed. Blood, like water or saline, is incompressible at *in vivo* pressures. Pressure builds up in the blood in the ventricular chambers and when the pressure reaches the pressure level in the pulmonary artery and aorta, the respective valves are pushed open. The ventricles then

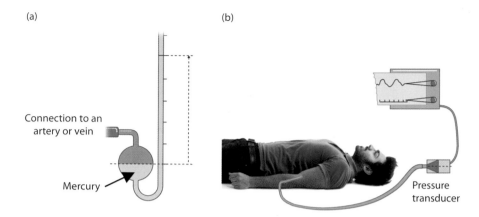

(a)   (b)

Connection to an
artery or vein

Mercury

Pressure
transducer

Figure 8.1 Blood pressure measuring devices. **(a)** Mercury-filled U-tube; **(b)** electronic pressure transducer. Pressure is measured in a hospital catheterization laboratory or intensive care unit with electronic pressure transducers as in **(b)** The tubing from an artery or vein **(b)** is filled with sterile saline. Blood pressure within, for instance, an artery pushes against the saline column in the tubing and the pressure is transmitted to the pressure transducer **(b)**. A pressure transducer **(b)** transforms pressure into voltage that is easily displayed and measured **(b)**. Direct connection to a mercury-filled system **(a)** has been used in the past, but is avoided because of concerns about mercury toxicity. Most clinical pressure measurement devices are spring-loaded or electronic sphygmomanometers. They are smaller and more convenient to use than a fluid column. Any pressure-measuring device can be called a manometer and "sphygmo-" refers to pulse. Blood pressure measuring devices are calibrated with a mercury column **(a)**.

push the blood into the great vessels, which already contain pressurized blood. This forces the vessels to expand and aortic and pulmonary artery pressure to increase further.

Kinetic energy, $(\rho v^2)/2$, appears because some pressure potential energy is transformed into movement of the blood through the great vessels; v, velocity, is distance moved per unit time. Density, ρ, is used to refer all calculations to a unit volume and mass of blood. In a person at rest, kinetic energy in the circulation relative to the other terms is small, approximately 3% to 5% of total energy, but it increases with, for instance, exercise. The last term, ρgh, appears here because gravity affects all mass in our world, including the mass of blood in blood vessels.

FLOW

If there is fluid flow in a system of tubes, the flow will occur from a point of higher total fluid energy to a point of lower total fluid energy. Water and a simple siphon can be used to illustrate this (Figure 8.2). In this simple model, there is no pump and the only energy to consider is gravitational potential energy. In this example, the flow of water is slow (low velocity) so that kinetic energy in the siphon is negligible.

The flow of fluid from 1 to 3 in Figure 8.2a and b depends only on the difference in total energy at 1 as compared with that at 3 and not on what happens to the tubing between the two points. The energy at point 1 is equal to the sum of atmospheric pressure + pressure potential energy due to the height of water above point 1. The energy at point 3 is equal only to atmospheric pressure. The difference in total energy from 1 to 3 is the pressure potential energy that moves fluid from 1 to 3.

Note also that at point 2 pressure is either higher (Figure 8.2a) or lower (Figure 8.2b) than at 1 or 3. However, it is the *pressure potential energy difference* between entry and exit points that determines flow in a siphon and not on the position of the fluid column in between.

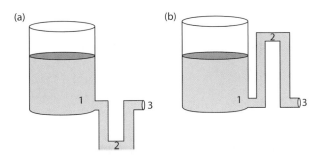

Figure 8.2 Siphon. The numbered locations and Fluid flow in a siphon is discussed in the text.

The siphon model is pertinent for the circulation because in the circulation the key energy term is pressure potential energy. As noted above, this energy derives from ATP split in ventricular myocyte sarcomeres. They develop force that produces ventricular pressure by squeezing on the blood within the ventricles. By splitting sarcomere crossbridge ATP and converting chemical into mechanical energy, the ventricles generate blood pressure and force a volume of blood into the aorta and pulmonary artery. That raises aortic and pulmonary artery blood pressure and blood then flows down a pressure gradient from the aorta, through the organ tissues, on to the veins and then the right atrium, and from the pulmonary artery through the lungs to the left atrium, just as in a siphon.

Consider the left ventricle and the peripheral circulation. Flow in the circulation acts like a siphon. As described in the preceding paragraph, the left ventricle generates blood pressure in the aorta. Blood pressure in the right atrium is very low. The difference in blood pressure from the aorta to the right atrium is large and the aorta is connected to the right atrium by blood vessel "tubing" that is filled with blood. Flow occurs from the aorta, through the organ blood vessels, to the right atrium. The same reasoning can be used to explain flow from the pulmonary artery, through the lungs, to the left atrium.

Blood has mass and is influenced by gravitational forces. This is true for both the arterial and venous parts of the circulation. In a standing person, venous blood pressure in the foot is higher than in the right atrium and arterial blood pressure in the foot is higher than in the aortic arch. Both pressures are higher due to the weight of the column of blood above the foot. But the physiological effects of gravity acting on the blood are most evident on the venous side of the circulation due to veins being much more compliant than arteries.

When a person is standing, gravity acting on the venous blood column results in an increase in venous blood pressure in the lower as compared with the upper body. The venous walls are compliant, the walls stretch easily and a significant volume of blood shifts from the upper to the lower body with standing. Gravity also increases blood pressure in the arteries of the lower body with standing, but arteries have relatively stiff walls that do not stretch as easily and there is no significant shift of arterial blood volume with standing. **There is a presentation of some effects of gravity on the circulation in the self-study module Transcapillary Exchange:** e **Starling Principle of Fluid Movement Across a Capillary Wall.**

The high compliance of the veins accounts for the fact that about two-thirds of the circulating blood volume resides in the venous system. As blood flows into the highly compliant venous system, the walls of the veins are stretched and the volume is then large. The systemic venous system is characterized by low blood pressure and large blood volume.

All the above brings us to some important concepts: (1) Blood moves through the circulation because of a pressure potential energy difference; the predominant energy difference from the aorta to the right atrium and from the pulmonary artery to the left atrium is the difference in pressure. (2) There is a significant shift of venous blood volume with postural changes.

Blood flow occurring because of pressure difference, like a siphon, is summarized in this formula:

$$Q = \frac{\bar{P}_1 - \bar{P}_2}{R}$$

Q is blood flow per unit time and R is vascular resistance. When considering the entire systemic circulation, Q is the same as cardiac output (CO), the volume of blood pumped per unit time, $\bar{P}_1$ is mean aortic pressure and $\bar{P}_2$ is mean right atrial pressure. Resistance in the systemic circulation resides mostly in the arterioles and is discussed in Chapter 11, Peripheral circulation. In the pulmonary circulation Q, again, is the cardiac output and the pressures of interest would be the mean pulmonary artery pressure, $\bar{P}_1$, and the mean left atrial pressure, $\bar{P}_2$.

BLOOD FLOW TYPES

LAMINAR FLOW

In Figure 8.3, the fluid column is flowing from left to right through the aorta. Blood pressure increase is generated by left ventricular contraction. Fluid in the center of the column is moving most rapidly. It is as if there are extremely thin concentric, onion-skin-like layers of fluid rubbing against each other with the central layer flowing the fastest (longest arrow in Figure 8.3) and the layer in contact with the wall not moving. When layered or laminar flow is present there is a velocity gradient from fast at the center to slow near the wall. Laminar flow is also called streamlined flow. The velocity wave front, the line joining the arrowheads, is parabolic (Figure 8.3).

Laminar or streamline flow exists because the internal rubbing mentioned above produces shear forces related to internal viscosity and results in an orderly, layered arrangement of flow velocity. Laminar flow is orderly and silent.

The most numerous formed elements of blood, the red blood cells, are nudged toward the center of the moving fluid column by the shear forces (Figure 8.3). There is a high concentration of red blood cells in blood, 4 to 5 million RBCs/μL, and their rubbing and bumping each other is a major contributor to normal blood viscosity.

e **The self-study module Cardiac Cycle: Heart Sounds and Murmurs contains a demonstration of laminar flow and presents its importance for clinical medicine.**

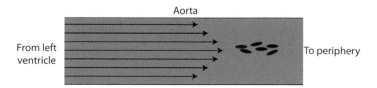

Figure 8.3 Laminar flow. Normal laminar or streamline flow in the aorta from left to right. Left ventricular contraction increases aortic blood pressure and flow occurs due to the higher pressure potential energy in the aorta than in the right atrium.

TURBULENT FLOW

In the self-study module Cardiac Cycle: Heart Sounds and Murmurs, there is a video demonstration of laminar and turbulent flow. An insoluble black dye is injected into the center of a stream of clear fluid flowing in a glass tube. The fluid flow rate is controlled and at the onset fluid flow is laminar or streamlined, with the black dye particles staying neatly in the center of the flowing fluid, like red blood cells in the aorta (Figure 8.3). Then, fluid flow velocity is gradually increased and when a critical velocity is reached the flow becomes turbulent. Turbulent flow is chaotic and disorganized rather than laminar and the black dye spreads throughout the cross-section of the tube due to the whorls and eddies of turbulence.

Once turbulence appears, some of the energy that would have produced an increase in forward flow now appears instead as chaotic whorls and eddies in the fluid column. **This is dramatically demonstrated in the video in the self-study module Cardiac Cycle: Heart Sounds and Murmurs.** In simple terms, when velocity, kinetic energy, reaches a high enough level to overcome the cohesive forces of internal fluid viscosity, organized laminar or streamlined flow changes to disorganized, chaotic, potentially noisy and less efficient turbulent flow.

In the self-study module Cardiac Cycle: Heart Sounds and Murmurs, there is a presentation of the effect of adding a constriction in the tube in which fluid is flowing. The pressure upstream of the constriction must be increased to keep the amount of fluid flowing per unit time through the constriction the same as before the constriction occurred. The amount of fluid flowing per unit time is unchanged, but velocity through the constriction is higher. This is discussed below.

Osborne Reynolds, a nineteenth century Irish engineer, first did the experiment with fluid flowing in a glass tube, described above. Reynolds showed that average velocity, tube diameter, and the viscosity and density of a liquid are crucial factors determining when turbulence appears. The Reynolds equation is

$$R_e = \frac{\bar{v} \, D \, \rho}{\eta}$$

where

R_e = Reynolds dimensionless number
$\bar{v}$ = Mean velocity, the velocity of forward fluid flow in cm/sec, averaged across the cross-section of laminar flow
D = Vessel diameter
ρ = Density of blood
η = Viscosity

Turbulence in the circulation appears when R_e increases and stays high. R_e must increase to approximately 2000 for turbulence to appear, but the actual value is influenced by the presence of pulsatile flow. Also, blood is a complex fluid and its viscosity varies with velocity. Blood viscosity is reduced at higher velocities because red blood cells tend to line up in the center of the stream and there is less rubbing and bumping of cells across the velocity wave front. Blood vessel architecture also influences the occurrence of turbulence, which is more likely to occur at branch points.

Laminar or streamline flow is well organized and it is silent. Turbulence is chaotic and noisy. The high velocity jet exiting a narrowing can result in turbulence. The turbulence occurs immediately downstream of the narrow area. One may be able to hear the noise with a stethoscope.

Such noise from a narrowed heart valve is called a "murmur" and from a narrowed artery or vein it is called a "bruit." **There are animated demonstrations of turbulence with heart valve narrowing in the self-study module Cardiac Cycle: Heart Sounds and Murmurs.**

There is another formula to consider that makes the Reynolds relationship clinically useful. The formula for velocity is

$$\bar{v} = \frac{Q}{A}$$

As noted above, $\bar{v}$ is the mean velocity of forward flow averaged over the flow wave front. A, the cross-sectional area of a valve orifice or a blood vessel, is calculated with the usual πr^2, and Q is the volume of blood flow per unit time. If this formula does not make immediate sense, try it with the accompanying units:

$$\bar{v}\left(\frac{cm}{sec}\right) = \frac{Q(cm^3/sec)}{A(cm^2)}$$

Notice that the units on the right side of the equation reduce to cm/sec, the units for linear velocity, and is then the same as the left side.

Both D and $\bar{v}$ are in the numerator in the Reynolds formula and A, area, is πr^2 or $\pi(D/2)^2$. Logic might lead one to conclude that as D decreases, for instance as an aortic valve narrows, $\bar{v}$ will increase and, therefore, R_e will not change. But R_e does increase in the presence of a narrow aortic valve and may increase enough that turbulence occurs in the aortic root (ascending aorta above the valve). The reason R_e increases in this instance is that $\bar{v}$ is inversely related to r^2, so $\bar{v}$ is an exponential function of r or D (2r) (Figure 8.4). When D decreases enough so that velocity rises significantly (Figure 8.4), R_e can increase enough for turbulence and noise to appear. The above suggests that with minimal narrowing of a heart valve, turbulence may be absent or minimal and a murmur will not be audible and that is the case.

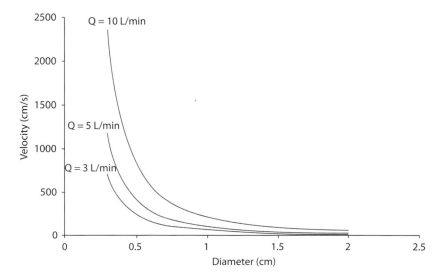

Figure 8.4 Velocity at a range of aortic valve areas and at three levels of cardiac output (Q). Normal aortic valve area is about 3 cm² with a diameter of about 2 cm.

Also, note the curves shift downward with decreasing Q (Figure 8.4). In a patient with, for instance, progressive aortic valve narrowing, cardiac output (Q) at rest will eventually decrease either due to severely compromised left ventricular heart muscle function or to the extremely high left ventricular pressure load. The patient will, of course, be severely disabled once Q is no longer adequate to meet the metabolic needs of the body at rest. As Q falls, velocity also falls (Figure 8.4). R_e may decrease enough so that turbulence lessens or disappears. In other words, late in the natural history of aortic valve narrowing, left ventricular function may be compromised enough that Q at rest is low and there may be little or no murmur. This emphasizes the fact that when applying a formula like $\bar{v} = (Q/A)$ in a clinical situation one must have information about two of the variables to draw conclusions about the third. **Learn more about this in the self-study module Cardiac Cycle: Heart Sounds and Murmurs.**

e

BLOOD FLOW VELOCITY IN THE CIRCULATION

This formula was used above to assess velocity through a narrow orifice, such as a narrow heart valve or a partial obstruction of a blood vessel:

$$\bar{v} = \frac{Q}{A}$$

Velocity of blood flow, v, relative to the amount of blood flow per unit time, Q, becomes important to consider when analyzing blood flow velocity throughout the body. Normal blood flow, cardiac output (Q), throughout the body at rest averages about 6 L/min in adults. The total cross-sectional area of the systemic capillary bed, the sum of πr^2 of all the individual capillaries, is the largest cross-sectional area in the systemic circulation, when compared with the aorta and its branches, the vena cavae and its branches, and so on (Figure 8.5). The circulation is a closed system, there are no alternative pathways for blood flow so the entire 6 L/min flows through the systemic capillary bed. The total 6 L/min of blood flow is divided among the millions of capillaries. Consequently, the blood flow and velocity are low in each capillary. The area (A) of the systemic capillary bed is the largest and the velocity of flow in this region is the smallest in the systemic circulation (Figure 8.5). Obviously, this is advantageous for gas and other exchange in the capillary beds. All the above comments also apply to the pulmonary circulation (Figure 8.5).

CLINICAL SIGNIFICANCE

The two formulas, R_e and $\bar{v} = (Q/A)$, are important to consider when murmurs or bruits occur in the circulation of a patient. For instance, R_e increases and turbulence can occur with the following changes in the circulatory system.

DIAMETER DECREASES

Narrowing of an artery, vein, or heart valve.

Q AND $\bar{v}$ INCREASE

The maternal circulating blood volume increases during pregnancy as total body metabolism increases with growth of the fetus. Maternal blood volume reaches a maximum at

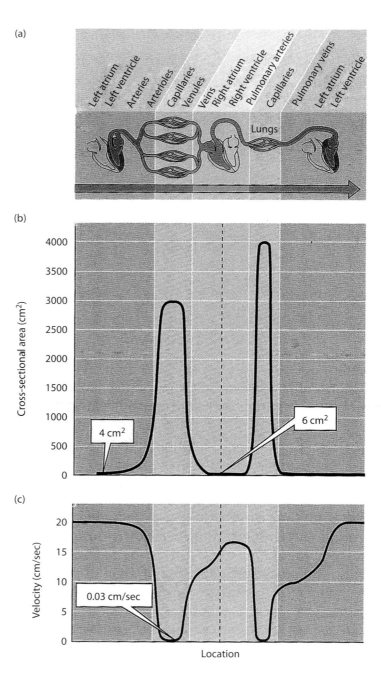

Figure 8.5 Cross-sectional area and velocity at locations in the circulation. Locations are illustrated at the top **(a)**. Total cross-sectional area is in **(b)**. Additionally, velocity of blood flow is in **(c)**. The enormous total cross-sectional area in the systemic and pulmonary capillaries results in very low velocity, since velocity (v) is inversely related to cross-sectional area (A): $v = (Q/A)$. Q is total flow or cardiac output, which is the same at all locations in the circulation. (Reprinted from *Medical Physiology*, 2nd ed., Boron WF, Copyright 2009, with permission from Elsevier.)

28–32 weeks of pregnancy. Cardiac output rises in parallel with the increasing blood volume. More blood volume increases ventricular filling and cardiac output (Q) (discussed below in Chapter 10, Ventricular function). The increase in Q increases $\bar{v}$ ($\bar{v} = Q/A$) and if there is enough of an increase, R_e increases to a level that results in turbulence. It is not unusual to hear a murmur that then disappears weeks after delivery when maternal cardiac output returns to pre-pregnancy levels.

LEAKING HEART VALVE

If Q and $\bar{v}$ through a leaking valve or defect is great enough, turbulence and a murmur can result.

DECREASED VISCOSITY (η)

If anemia is severe enough to decrease η enough, the increased Reynolds number can result in turbulence in many blood vessels. There are likely to be multiple bruits and a systolic murmur.

Density of the blood, ρ, does not change significantly with various alterations of blood and changes in ρ are not likely to contribute to the development of turbulence in clinical problems.

Cardiac cycle, heart sounds, and murmurs

9

THE CIRCULATION

The right atrium (RA) receives blood low in oxygen from the vena cavae and delivers blood to the right ventricle (RV) (Figure 9.1). The RV pumps blood into the pulmonary artery (PA). The left atrium (LA) receives oxygenated blood from the pulmonary veins and blood then flows into the left ventricle (LV). The LV pumps blood into the aorta (Ao) (Figure 9.1).

CARDIAC VALVES

The atrioventricular valves are the tricuspid and mitral valves. The tricuspid valve allows one-way flow from the RA to the RV and the mitral valve from the LA to the LV. The semilunar valves are the pulmonic and aortic valves. The pulmonic valve allows only one-way flow from the RV to the PA and the aortic valve from the LV to the Ao.

All four valves open when pressure on the upstream* side begins to exceed pressure on the downstream side. The atrioventricular valves close when ventricular pressure increases and ventricular blood is thrust back toward the atrioventricular valve. The semilunar valves close when forward flow in the pulmonary artery and aorta ceases and begins to reverse as the ventricles begin to relax.

ATRIAL AND VENTRICULAR PHASES OF THE CARDIAC CYCLE

Left-sided events are depicted in Figures 9.2 and 9.3. Pressures in the right heart chambers are normally much lower than in the left. Other than pressure levels, the timing and characteristics of events in the right heart are like those in the left heart. The following description of the cardiac cycle will start at the end of diastole when atrial depolarization occurs.

ATRIAL SYSTOLE AT THE END OF DIASTOLE

"Systole" is derived from a Greek word for contraction. After the sinoatrial (SA) node depolarizes, depolarization then spreads throughout the atrial musculature and atrial wall contraction

---

* Think of the bloodstream as a river. For instance, upstream from the mitral valve are the left atrium, pulmonary veins, and so on. The left ventricle, aorta, and so on are downstream from the mitral valve.

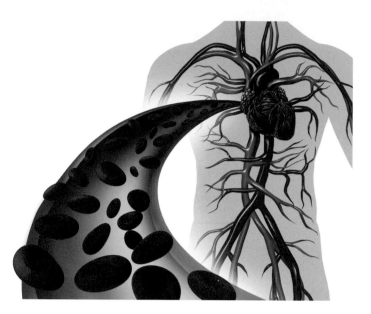

Figure 9.1 The circulation.

occurs. The tricuspid and mitral valves have been open all through filling and remain open (Figure 9.2). Atrial muscle contraction (Figure 9.2, atrial systole) increases blood pressure in the atria, in the veins entering the atria, and in the ventricles. Note the left atrial "a" pressure wave in Figure 9.3. A similar "a" wave occurs in the right atrium.

Right and left atrial systole occur at the end of ventricular filling (Figure 9.2). Atrial systole results in a small push of blood from the atria into the ventricles called the atrial "kick." The contribution of the atrial kick to ventricular filling is small, but becomes more significant:

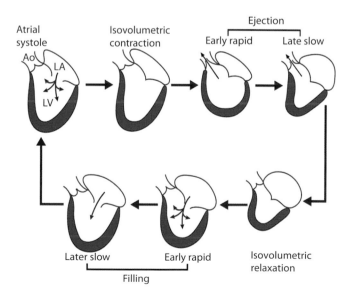

Figure 9.2 Cardiac cycle events in the left heart. Filling, after early rapid and later slow filling, concludes with atrial systole and the atrial kick. This is discussed in the text.

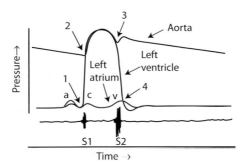

Figure 9.3 Cardiac cycle. Mitral valve closes after 1, aortic valve opens at 2, aortic valve closes at 3, and mitral valve opens at 4. S1 is the first heart sound and S2 the second.

- When heart rate is high and time for ventricular filling is short, such as in exercise.
- In a patient in severe heart failure, where the extra ventricular filling becomes important for adequate ventricular function.

ISOVOLUMETRIC CONTRACTION

Depolarization spreads over the atria and then is delayed in the atrioventricular node. Next it enters the bundle of His and the bundle branches, then spreads throughout the ventricles. Ventricular muscle contraction begins and force develops in the ventricular wall. The contracting ventricular wall squeezes the blood within the left ventricular chamber. Blood pressure within the ventricles starts to increase as ventricular blood is thrust back toward the atrioventricular valves. The tricuspid and mitral valve leaflets are pushed close (Figure 9.2, isovolumetric contraction and 1 in Figure 9.3).

After the mitral valve closes, left ventricular pressure continues to increase (Figures 9.2 and 9.3, from 1 to 2). The mitral valve closes immediately after 1 and the aortic valve will not be pushed open until 2 (Figure 9.3). The left ventricular pressure increase from 1 to 2 (Figure 9.3) is termed isovolumetric because the mitral and aortic valves are closed, blood in the ventricles cannot move, and ventricular volume remains constant. The same occurs in the right ventricle at close to the same time.

The "c" wave in the left atrial pressure tracing (Figure 9.3) during isovolumetric contraction is related to a small amount of bulging of the closed mitral valve into the blood-filled left atrial cavity. The bulging is due to the isovolumetric left ventricular pressure increase causing slight ballooning of the closed mitral valve. A similar c wave occurs in the right atrial pressure tracing for the same reason. There is ballooning of the closed atrioventricular valves. They do not normally open at this time.

EJECTION

When ventricular pressure rises to and begins to exceed that in the aorta and pulmonary artery, the semilunar valves open (Figure 9.2, early rapid ejection; 2 in Figure 9.3). Rapid ejection of blood from the ventricles into the pulmonary artery and aorta begins. Ventricular volume rapidly decreases.

Blood flow out of the ventricles is initially rapid (Figure 9.2, early rapid ejection). Left ventricular and aortic pressure rise to a maximal level (Figure 9.3). Pressure increases simultaneously in the left ventricle and the aorta (Figure 9.3) because the aortic valve is open. The amount of blood ejected from the left ventricle into the aorta during early rapid ejection exceeds the amount leaving the arterial system through the arterioles (peripheral runoff). The aortic volume increases, the proximal aortic wall is stretched, and aortic and left ventricular pressures increase.

Aortic and left ventricular pressures then simultaneously fall from their maximum (Figure 9.3) for two reasons:

- Left ventricular ejection begins to decline (Figure 9.2, later slow ejection). Left ventricular ejection slows because of relaxation of the ventricular myocytes. Relaxation is related to Ca^{2+} uptake by the sarcoplasmic reticulum. **This is presented in the self-study module Clinical Heart Muscle Physiology, Part 1: Activation and Relaxation.**

- Blood is leaving the aorta and its branches, flowing through the arterioles (peripheral runoff) and entering the capillary beds around the body. During later slower ejection, the amount of peripheral runoff exceeds the amount ejected into the aorta by the left ventricle. Aortic blood volume decreases, the proximal aortic walls are less stretched, and aortic and left ventricular pressures fall (Figure 9.3).

Similar events are occurring in the right ventricle and pulmonary artery.

Ventricular relaxation continues. Ventricular ejection further slows (Figure 9.2, late slow ejection) and finally ceases. The column of blood in the aorta immediately proximal to the aortic valve momentarily moves back toward the aortic valve. This part of the aorta is called the aortic root and the movement of the aortic root blood column back toward the valve is brief. It is brief because the moment the blood column moves back toward the valve, the aortic valve promptly closes (Figure 9.2, transition from late slow ejection to isovolumic relaxation and Figure 9.3, valve closure occurs at point 3). Similarly, pulmonary artery flow reverses and the pulmonary valve closes.

When the aortic valve closes, the column of blood in the aortic root bounces against the closed valve. The aortic root blood column, the aortic valve, and the aortic root wall vibrate. The vibrations are manifest in the aortic pressure tracing as a notch and rebound (Figure 9.3, notch in the aortic pressure tracing at point 3). This notch is called the dicrotic notch or incisura. There is a similar notch in a pulmonary artery pressure tracing.

ISOVOLUMETRIC RELAXATION

Isovolumetric relaxation begins as soon as the pulmonary and aortic valves close (Figure 9.2, isovolumetric relaxation and Figure 9.3, from point 3 to 4). The atrioventricular valves remain shut because ventricular pressures are still higher than atrial pressures (Figure 9.2, isovolumetric relaxation). All the valves are now shut. Ventricular muscle relaxation continues and intraventricular pressures decrease (Figure 9.3, left ventricular pressure decrease from 3 to 4).

DIASTOLIC FILLING

The tricuspid and mitral valves open (Figure 9.2, early rapid filling and Figure 9.3 at point 4) as soon as ventricular pressure drops to and then below the level of atrial pressure. The pulmonary and aortic valves remain shut (Figure 9.2).

The atria have been isolated from the ventricles and filling during isovolumetric contraction, ejection, and isovolumetric relaxation. The atrioventricular valves remain shut throughout ventricular ejection because ventricular pressure is higher than atrial pressure. Pulmonary artery mean pressure is higher than left atrial mean pressure during this time and the left atrial wall is compliant. Blood flows through the pulmonary circulation much like a siphon from pulmonary artery to left atrium and left atrial filling results in a rise in atrial pressure called the v wave (Figure 9.3). Aorta to right atrium blood flow occurs for similar reasons and right atrial filling also results in a v wave.

At the conclusion of isovolumetric relaxation, the atria are engorged with blood and their walls are stretched (Figure 9.2). When the atrioventricular valves open, ventricular filling is initially *very* rapid (Figure 9.2, early rapid filling). This is a passive transfer of blood from atria to ventricles driven by elastic forces in the atrial walls—no muscle contraction is involved. The filling is aided by rapid ventricular relaxation continuing during the beginning of the diastolic filling period—note the decrease in ventricular pressure after 4 in Figure 9.3. The ventricles develop a small amount of suction at this time that aids filling. The initial increase in ventricular volume is rapid and about 80% of ventricular filling occurs during early rapid filling.

After early rapid ventricular filling, the heart functions as if composed of two chambers, a right and left. The right atrium and ventricle fill from the vena cavae and the left atrium and ventricle fill from the pulmonary veins. Filling is now slower than initial rapid filling and filling lasts until the onset of the next cardiac cycle (Figures 9.2 and 9.3 from point 4 to point 1).

As noted above, about 80% of ventricular filling occurs during early rapid filling. Another 5% of filling occurs during later slow filling until atrial systole. Atrial kick contributes the remaining, approximately 15% of filling. The diastolic filling period then consists of three phases: early rapid filling, slower filling and atrial kick.

NORMAL INTRAVASCULAR PRESSURES IN PEOPLE

Location	Pressure (mm Hg)	
	Average value	Normal range
Right atrium	3 (mean)	2–7 (mean)
Right ventricle peak systolic	25	15–30
End-diastolic	4	1–7
Pulmonary artery peak systolic	25	15–30
Diastolic	9	4–12
Left atrium	8 (mean)	2–12 (mean)
Left ventricle peak systolic	130	90–140
End-diastolic	8	5–12
Aorta systolic	130	90–140
Diastolic	85	60–90

HEART SOUNDS

FIRST HEART SOUND, S1

S1 is low in frequency and occurs through most of isovolumetric contraction (Figure 9.3). At the onset of ventricular contraction, blood in the ventricles is pushed toward the atrioventricular valves. The atrioventricular valves are pushed closed and this results in the first prominent component of S1, mitral and tricuspid valve closure. The vibrating valves, oscillations in the blood in the ventricles, and vibrations of the ventricular wall all contribute to the long low frequency S1.

SECOND HEART SOUND, S2

As noted earlier, the aortic valve closes at the end of ejection when the column of blood in the aortic root begins to move back toward the valve. Similar events occur in the pulmonary artery and pulmonary valve. Vibrations occur in the taut valve leaflets, the vessel wall adjacent to the valve, and in the suddenly decelerating blood column. These oscillations result in the notch and rebound in pressure recordings from the aorta or pulmonary artery, the dicrotic notch or incisura, that is coincident with S2 and is discussed above (Figure 9.3, point 3).

S2 is higher in frequency than the first sound, in other words, it is "snappier." Normally, pulmonary valve closure (P2) is later than aortic valve closure (A2). The delay of P2 increases during inspiration (Figure 9.4). This "splitting" of the second sound into an aortic component followed by a pulmonary artery component is audible during normal inspiration. The splitting is not pictured in Figure 9.3.

The inspiratory S2 split occurs because intrathoracic pressure drops further below atmospheric during inspiration. The intrathoracic pressure is the pressure inside the chest, but outside the lungs, heart, and intrathoracic blood vessels. This decrease in pressure below atmospheric pressure (suction) outside the heart and intrathoracic blood vessels affects these structures because their size depends on the pressure difference across their walls, the inside minus the external pressure. This pressure difference is called the transmural pressure, P_t. As an example, P_t for the pulmonary artery is blood pressure within the pulmonary artery minus the pressure within the thorax external to the pulmonary artery, the intrathoracic pressure. This fits with the definition of P_t as the pressure internal to a hollow structure (P_i) minus the external pressure (P_e).

$$P_t = P_i - P_e$$

Consider the pulmonary artery and its major branches external to the lung, the extrapulmonic pulmonary arterial vessels. Intrathoracic pressure is the P_e and blood pressure inside the extrapulmonic pulmonary arteries is P_i. As intrathoracic pressure (P_e) decreases with inspiration, P_i does not significantly change and P_t increases. The result is an increase in diameter of the extrapulmonic pulmonary arterial vessels. This increases the capacity (capacitance, Figure 9.5) of extrapulmonic pulmonary arterial blood vessels. This increased pulmonary arterial capacity in inspiration permits forward blood flow in the pulmonary artery to last longer than in expiration. Think of this as "more room" for blood flow. During inspiration the duration of pulmonary artery blood flow is longer, the reversal of blood flow in the pulmonary artery is delayed, pulmonary valve closure is delayed, and P2 occurs later (Figures 9.4 and 9.5).

More room or capacity in the extrapulmonic pulmonary arteries during inspiration suggests there is more blood in those vessels during inspiration and there is. The intrathoracic negative

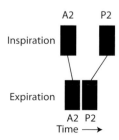

Figure 9.4 Bar diagram of second heart sound splitting. A2 refers to the aortic component and P2 to the pulmonic component of S2.

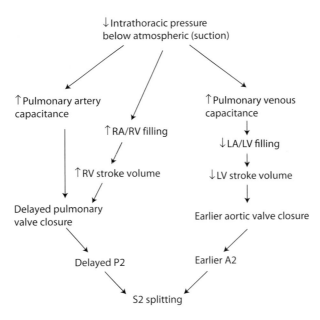

Figure 9.5 Second heart sound splitting mechanisms. RA = right atrium, RV = right ventricle, LA = left atrium, LV = left ventricle, P2 = pulmonic component of the second heart sound (S2), and A2 = aortic component of S2.

pressure or suction created during inspiration is the P_e, the intrathoracic pressure external to the right heart structures, including the thoracic portion of the cavae, right atrium, and right ventricle. The increased P_t in those structures draws systemic venous blood into the right heart during inspiration. Right ventricular filling and stroke volume increase (Figure 9.5). The normal splitting of S2 then is the interplay of changes in extrapulmonic pulmonary arterial capacitance with changes in right heart filling and stroke volume (Figure 9.5).

Another result of the decrease below atmospheric pressure in the thorax during inspiration is an increase in extrapulmonic pulmonary venous capacitance (Figure 9.5). The pulmonary veins external to the lungs are thin-walled and very compliant. They hold more blood during inspiration and less blood then flows to the left atrium and ventricle (Figure 9.5). Left ventricular filling is reduced, stroke volume is less, ejection ends earlier, aortic valve closure is earlier (Figure 9.5), and A2 occurs slightly earlier. The delay in pulmonary valve closure during inspiration contributes much more to S2 splitting than the earlier closure of the aortic valve (Figure 9.4).

THIRD HEART SOUND, S3

During early rapid ventricular filling (Figure 9.2), a low pitched third heart sound may be heard in normal young people, below the age of 30–40 years (Figure 9.6). The likely mechanisms include vibrations in the ventricular wall related to the rapid filling. An S3 can be normal or abnormal.

A third heart sound may be audible at the apex when:

- Blood flow rate and the rate of ventricular filling are high.
  Examples: anemia, fever, or pregnancy.
- Either ventricle is dilated, there is increased ventricular wall stiffness, or both.
  Example: heart disease accompanied by abnormally increased ventricular filling and ventricular hypertrophy. Obviously, this would be an abnormal S3.

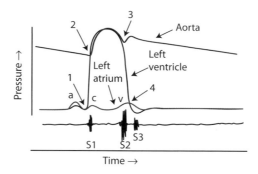

Figure 9.6 Third heart sound (S3). S1 and S2 are the first and second heart sounds, respectively.

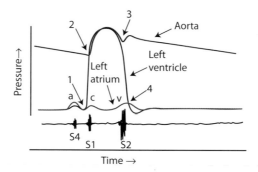

Figure 9.7 Fourth heart sound (S4). S1 and S2 are the first and second heart sounds, respectively.

FOURTH HEART SOUND, S4

A sound can occur coincident with atrial contraction (Figure 9.7) and result from the atrial "kick" in the presence of a stiffer than normal ventricle. The sound is likely generated by vibrations of the ventricular wall and the blood in the ventricular lumen. Ventricular hypertrophy with increased ventricular wall stiffness is the typical situation that produces an S4. It is not heard in normal people.

MURMURS DURING THE CARDIAC CYCLE

Acquired or congenital valvular heart disease occurs when a valve orifice becomes narrowed (valvular stenosis) or when a valve does not close completely (valvular insufficiency or regurgitation). A noise or murmur occurs in the presence of valvular stenosis because of turbulence immediately downstream of the defect. The turbulence is upstream of a leaking valve. **The location of turbulence with a heart valve defect and other features of murmurs are presented in the self-study module Cardiac Cycle: Heart Sounds and Murmurs. The module includes animations of streamline flow, turbulence, and murmurs.**

There are two definitions of systole and diastole. The clinical definition is an outgrowth of classifying murmurs and began early in the use of stethoscopes. The physiological definition of systole and diastole is based on more recent hemodynamic measurements and an understanding of myocardial mechanics. The definitions are as follows:

1. Clinical systole consists of the events from S1 to S2 and include isovolumetric contraction and ejection. Clinical diastole is from S2 to the next S1 and includes isovolumetric relaxation and the diastolic filling period.
2. Physiological systole consists of events from the closure of the atrioventricular valves to the valves opening and includes isovolumetric contraction, ejection, and isovolumetric relaxation. Physiological diastole consists of the diastolic filling period.

Murmurs are named using the clinical definition of systole and diastole and that is what will be used throughout the following discussion.

The aortic valve will be used for the examples in the following discussion of murmurs. Murmurs related to defects in the other valves can be analyzed using the principles presented here. **There is a more extensive discussion of murmurs and heart sounds in the self-study module Cardiac Cycle: Heart Sounds and Murmurs.**

SYSTOLIC MURMUR

If the aortic valve orifice is narrow (aortic valvular stenosis), turbulence occurs in the root of the aorta during ejection. If the turbulence generates vibrations with enough energy, the turbulence can be audible as a systolic murmur. The murmur can be recorded (phonocardiogram) with a microphone placed on the chest (Figure 9.8).

The murmur of aortic valvular stenosis cannot begin until flow starts through the narrowed aortic valve orifice. The murmur cannot start until ejection begins at the end of isovolumetric contraction. S1 is heard during isovolumetric contraction and should be audible and normal since the murmur does not start until the end of isovolumetric contraction. The murmur should end toward the end of ejection when flow out of the left ventricle into the aorta slows. With slower flow during later, slower ejection, there is reduced velocity and turbulence. The second heart sound should be audible. Similar reasoning can be used for the murmur of pulmonary valvular stenosis. **There is a complete presentation of the characteristics of this type of murmur in the self-study module Cardiac Cycle: Heart Sounds and Murmurs.**

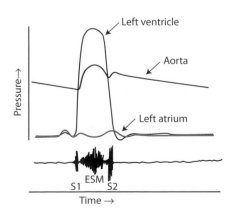

Figure 9.8 Left ventricular and atrial pressure, aortic pressure, and the phonocardiogram in aortic valvular stenosis. S1 is the first heart sound and S2 the second. ESM = ejection systolic murmur.

A systolic murmur can be present without a defect of the heart or great vessels (see section on turbulent flow in Chapter 8, How the Circulation Works). Such a so-called "innocent" or "flow" or "physiologic" murmur is typically systolic.

DIASTOLIC MURMUR

If the aortic valve does not close tightly, blood will leak into the ventricle from the aorta during isovolumetric relaxation at the onset of diastole. The murmur of aortic valvular insufficiency (also called aortic valvular regurgitation) begins with A2 and lasts through a portion of diastole (Figure 9.9). A2 may be diminished or absent when the valve deformity limits aortic valve leaflet movement. P2 is often obscured by the murmur.

Note: With the diastolic murmur of aortic valvular insufficiency, the turbulence is in the left ventricle immediately upstream of the aortic valve. An ejection systolic murmur (Figure 9.9) may be present if the aortic valvular insufficiency is severe enough. It is likely due to the large diastolic filling of the left ventricle from the regurgitant flow plus the usual filling from the left atrium. The left ventricular wall is stretched more and there is a large total stroke volume. The large flow out of the left ventricle during ejection results in high velocity and increases R_e. If R_e increases enough there will be systolic ejection turbulence.

Here is how to figure out when in the cardiac cycle a murmur will likely occur for a specific valve defect. For example, consider mitral valvular stenosis (narrowing of the mitral valve orifice). This is a defect in which the valve does not fully open. The steps to define the timing of the murmur are

- First, have clearly in mind when in the cardiac cycle the valve is supposed to be fully open or completely closed. The mitral valve should be fully open during the entire diastolic filling period, but in mitral valvular stenosis, the mitral valve cannot fully open.
- Second, pinpoint the part of the cardiac cycle where the valve malfunction will be manifest. The mitral valve is supposed to open fully at the end of isovolumetric relaxation and the beginning of filling of the left ventricle. It is supposed to stay open throughout the diastolic filling period.

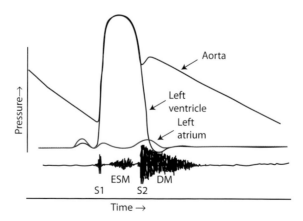

Figure 9.9 Left ventricular and atrial pressure, aortic pressure, and the phonocardiogram in aortic valvular insufficiency/regurgitation. S1 is the first heart sound. S2 is the second heart sound and is obscured by the diastolic murmur, DM. ESM = ejection systolic murmur.

- Obviously, flow through the mitral valve orifice normally occurs when it is open. If it is narrow and cannot fully open, that is when a murmur will occur. Therefore, the murmur of mitral stenosis can be present all through the diastolic filling period. The murmur must end with S1. Closure of the mitral valve ends flow across the valve and the murmur.

There is a detailed presentation of mitral valvular stenosis and other valve defects in the self-study module Cardiac Cycle: Hearts Sounds and Murmurs.

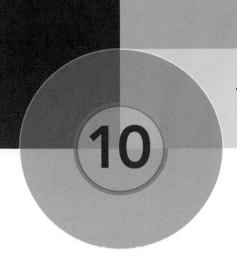

Ventricular function

Ventricular function is best understood after studying heart muscle function. Preload, contractility, and afterload are the major determinants of ventricular function and are functional parameters based on ventricular myocyte mechanical properties. **The accompanying three-part self-study module, Clinical Cardiac Muscle Physiology, explores heart muscle physiology and is designed to facilitate the study of ventricular function**. You will be at a disadvantage if you do not do the module before considering ventricular function.

PRELOAD

CHANGES IN VENTRICULAR FILLING

The volume of ventricular ejection, the stroke volume, is partly determined by the amount of preceding diastolic filling. The meaning of the relationship in Figure 10.1 is that the more a ventricle fills, the more it ejects. Ventricular filling stretches ventricular wall myocytes. With less filling, stroke volume is less and with increased filling, stroke volume increases. This is the Frank–Starling law of the heart. The law is another way of stating that the length of ventricular wall myocytes at the end of filling, the preload, is one major determinant of ventricular function. An increase in ventricular end-diastolic volume is accompanied by an increase in resting myocyte length and resting sarcomere length. **Preload and the effect of resting myocyte length on cardiac muscle function is presented in the self-study module Clinical Heart Muscle Physiology, Part 2: Muscle Mechanics Made Easy**.

Stroke volume (SV) (Figure 10.1) and cardiac output (CO) are relatively simple measures of ventricular performance used in the following discussion. Stroke volume is the amount of blood ejected by a ventricle during a single cardiac cycle. Cardiac output is the amount of blood pumped by the heart per minute and is the product of the stroke volume (amount ejected per cardiac cycle) and the heart rate (cardiac cycles per minute).

$$CO\left(\frac{mL\ blood}{min}\right) = SV\left(\frac{mL\ blood}{beat}\right) \times HR\left(\frac{beats}{min}\right)$$

Representative factors that result in increased or decreased ventricular filling and end-diastolic volume are noted below the horizontal axis in Figure 10.1. The amount of ventricular filling sets the end-diastolic volume and length of ventricular wall myocytes. Ventricular

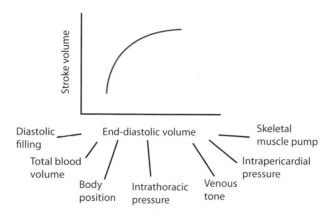

Figure 10.1 Frank–Starling law of the heart. A representative sample of influences on end-diastolic volume are arrayed below the horizontal axis.

filling and the Frank–Starling law are important in the normal heart for beat-by-beat regulation of stroke volume and for accommodation of the ventricles to the amount of circulating blood volume.

Reduced total blood volume becomes clinically important, for instance, in dehydration or blood loss. Changes in ventricular filling due to changes in intrathoracic pressure during normal respiration were presented earlier in the discussion of S2 splitting (Chapter 9, Cardiac cycle, heart sounds and murmurs). Stroke volume varies with respiration, but is the same in the two ventricles when averaged over multiple respiratory cycles. The skeletal muscle pump refers to the intermittent compression of lower extremity deep veins with cyclic muscle contraction during walking or running. The lower extremity deep veins are surrounded by muscle and have valves. Compression of the veins moves venous blood toward the heart through the valves that are pushed open. With relaxation, the venous blood starts to move backward, but the valves close. Thus, with lower extremity rhythmic exercise deep venous blood is pumped toward the right atrium.

The pericardial sac normally contains a small amount of serous fluid under negligible pressure for lubrication of the sac internal surfaces. If, for example, pericardial inflammation, pericarditis, results in excess sac fluid accumulation, sac pressure can increase to an extent that limits ventricular filling. Even the normal pericardial sac acts to prevent excessive ventricular filling.

Body position influences end-diastolic volume because of the effects of gravity. In upright posture, there is a shift of venous blood to the lower body and reduced ventricular end-diastolic volume. This is discussed in the section on arterial neural baroreceptors in Chapter 12, Circulatory Controls. **The effects of gravity on the circulation are presented in the self-study module Transcapillary Fluid Exchange.**

PRESSURE-VOLUME LOOP

Ventricular pressure and volume during the cardiac cycle can be plotted to create a pressure-volume loop (Figure 10.2). Pressure-volume loops are useful to evaluate ventricular function and the area of the loop is a measure of ventricular work.

The end of the diastolic filling period and closure of the mitral valve is at point A in the cardiac cycle (Figure 10.2). The end-diastolic pressure is low in a normal ventricle and the volume is large so A in the pressure-volume loop figure is at a high volume, low pressure point (Figure 10.2). Pressure rises from A to B without a change in volume during the isovolumetric

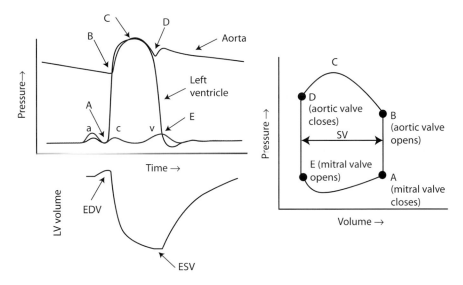

Figure 10.2 Construction of a pressure-volume loop. EDV is end-diastolic volume and ESV is end-systolic volume. SV is stroke volume.

contraction phase of the cardiac cycle (Figure 10.2). At B, the aortic valve opens and ventricular ejection occurs from B to D as left ventricular pressure rises to a maximum at C.

The aortic valve closes at D and the isovolumetric relaxation phase of the cardiac cycle, D to E, begins. At E, the mitral valve opens (Figure 10.2) and ventricular filling proceeds from E to A. Ventricular relaxation finishes with a further drop in pressure after E. (Figure 10.2). The horizontal distance in the pressure-volume loop from point A to D (Figure 10.2) is the stroke volume.

A ventricular pressure-volume loop changes with an increase in preload based on the Frank–Starling law of the heart discussed earlier (Figure 10.1). An increase in ventricular volume from A to A′ stretches ventricular wall sarcomeres, improves function, and increases stroke volume (Figure 10.3). D shifts to the right to D′ with more filling and to D″ with additional filling. The stroke volume as measured by the horizontal distance from A to D increases to A′ to D′ and further increases to A″ to D″.

The end-systolic pressure-volume points D, D′, and D″ define a linear relationship, the end-systolic pressure volume relationship (ESPVR) (Figure 10.3). The slope of the ESPVR defines an inotropic state or level of contractility. The fact that D, D′, and D″ all fall on the same ESPVR indicates contractility has not been changed by changes in filling. In this example, stroke volume increased due to an increase in filling, not an increase in contractility. The ESPVR intersects the horizontal axis at close to zero, which is beyond the left edge of the graph.

Contractility is presented in the self-study module Clinical Heart Muscle Physiology, Part 3: Cardiac Contractility.

e

CONTRACTILITY

VENTRICULAR FUNCTION CURVES

Ventricular function cannot be explained in all circumstances with one Starling curve. For instance, changes in sympathetic stimulation can change ventricular function without a change

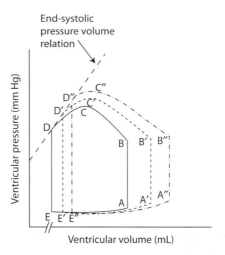

Figure 10.3 Pressure volume loops and end-systolic pressure-volume relation with changes in ventricular filling. As described in the text and shown in Figure 10.2, stroke volume (SV) is the horizontal distance from A to D. SV is increased as end-diastolic volume increases to A' and A".

in end-diastolic volume. A change in function without a change in end-diastolic volume only can happen with shift to a different Starling or ventricular function curve (Figure 10.4).

Sympathetic stimulation of heart muscle occurs in two ways:

- Release of norepinephrine at cardiac sympathetic nerve endings.
- Mostly epinephrine and some norepinephrine released from the adrenal medulla, borne by the bloodstream to the coronary circulation and carried in the coronary blood to the cardiac myocytes.

Neurotransmitter and hormonal catecholamines interact with β receptors on the surface of myocytes. This interaction with myocyte β receptors initiates a cascade of intracellular events that results in an increase in the myocardial contractile state. The effects involve increased inward Ca^{2+} movement through sarcolemmal L-type Ca^{2+} channels, cAMP and increased

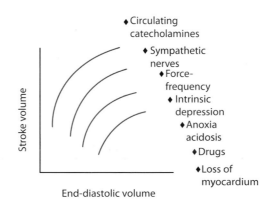

Figure 10.4 A family of ventricular function curves. Some of the influences on ventricular contractility are listed.

Ca^{2+}-induced release of Ca^{2+} from the sarcoplasmic reticulum terminal cisternae. The resulting increase in ventricular function can occur with no change in end-diastolic volume and cannot be explained by a single ventricular function curve.

Each curve in Figure 10.4 characterizes the relationship of end-diastolic volume with ventricular performance for a contractile or inotropic state of ventricular myocardium. A normal ventricle moves among the curves mostly due to moment-to-moment changes in ventricular muscle contractile or inotropic state secondary to more or less sympathetic stimulation. As discussed earlier, the level of function along one curve is determined by the amount of ventricular filling, the end-diastolic volume.

Some factors that increase or decrease contractility or the inotropic state are noted in Figure 10.4. Force-frequency in Figure 10.4 refers to treppe, discussed in the self-study module Clinical Cardiac Muscle Physiology Part 3. Cardiac Contractility. The effects of force-frequency (heart rate) on ventricular contractility are small relative to the effects of sympathetic stimulation and circulating catecholamines. **Catecholamine effects on contractility are also discussed in the Clinical Cardiac Muscle Physiology Part 3 module.** Intrinsic depression refers to depressed contractility that occurs in some types of ventricular dysfunction. Myocardial infarction resulting from lack of coronary blood flow to a portion of a ventricle is the most common example of loss of myocardium mentioned in Figure 10.4. **Myocardial infarction and resulting ventricular dysfunction is discussed in the self-study module Myocardial Infarction and Chronic Heart Failure.** Many drugs depress contractility, including certain anesthetic agents. There are also drugs that increase contractility. Anoxia and acidosis are obvious examples of changes in the chemical environment of myocytes that can adversely affect their function.

PRESSURE-VOLUME LOOP AND CONTRACTILITY

An increase in contractility is expected to result in more ventricular force development and faster and more myocyte shortening. The ventricle should empty more and develop more pressure.

As an example, suppose sympathetic stimulation of a ventricle increases. Remember, every cardiac myocyte is innervated by sympathetic nerves. The increased sympathetic stimulation results in an increase in myocyte contractility. Function shifts to a higher ventricular function curve and stroke volume likely increases (Figure 10.4). Note the leftward shift of the

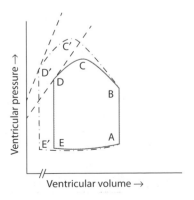

Figure 10.5 Ventricular pressure-volume loops with increased contractility. Points A and B are the same for both loops. The broken line loop resulted after an increase in contractility.

end-systolic pressure-volume point D leftward to D' onto a new, steeper ESPVR (Figure 10.5). The ESPVRs in Figure 10.5 intersect the horizontal axis at close to zero off the left side of the graph, just as in Figure 10.3.

This type of ESPVR shift is one measure of an increase in ventricular contractility. Stroke volume is increased as evidenced by the increase in the horizontal distance AD to AD'. In this portrayal, there is no change in end-diastolic volume, A.

The end-systolic pressure-volume point D has shifted to D' on a new steeper end-systolic pressure-volume relation, an indication of an increase in contractility (Figure 10.5). Here the stroke volume has increased due to an increase in contractility, but with no change in the extent of ventricular filling (preload).

AFTERLOAD

The afterload is the load on a ventricle during contraction. It is called "afterload" because it is the load on the ventricles after contraction begins. A precise measure of ventricular afterload involves measuring ventricular wall stress or force, since wall force is what myocytes must work with during pressure development and shortening. Intraventricular pressure and chamber radius must be measured to estimate wall stress. Fortunately, aortic pressure is more easily measured and serves as an index of the level of afterload for the left ventricle and for the right ventricle it is pulmonary artery pressure.

Normal left ventricular afterload increases with increases in aortic systolic blood pressure. For instance, afterload increases with a reflex increase in peripheral vascular resistance with skin vasoconstriction in cold ambient temperatures. Aortic systolic pressure increases and a sequence of events occurs in a normal heart that mostly preserves left ventricular stroke volume (Figure 10.6):

- The increased load on left ventricular myocytes causes them to shorten less and more slowly in the first few beats after aortic pressure increases. **The effects of load on myocyte shortening is presented in the self-study module Clinical Cardiac Muscle Physiology, Part 2: Muscle Mechanics Made Easy.**
- Stroke volume decreases in those first few beats. This is not shown in Figure 10.6.
- More blood remains in the left ventricle at the end of ejection. In other words, end-systolic volume increases.

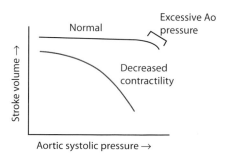

Figure 10.6 Stroke volume response to changes in aortic systolic pressure in normal ventricles and with decreased contractility. Ao = aortic.

- The usual amount of filling of the left ventricle adds to the increased blood left in the ventricle (the increased end-systolic volume) and the end-diastolic volume increases.
- The resultant increase in end-diastolic volume returns the stroke volume almost to where it was before aortic pressure increased.

In summary then, the steady state response to an increase in afterload in a normal left ventricle is an increase in both end-diastolic and end-systolic volume, with a slight decrease in steady state stroke volume (Figure 10.6). In a normal ventricle, the stroke volume is close to unchanged when aortic pressure changes (Figure 10.6).

The preservation of steady state stroke volume when ventricular afterload increases can be described using pressure-volume loops (Figure 10.7). The horizontal distance A′ to D′ is slightly less than that for A to D. End-diastolic volume increased from A to A′ as did end-systolic volume from D to D′. ESPVR does not shift so the response to the increased afterload is not due to a change in contractility, but rather to more filling. Normally stroke volume decreases very little with pressure increases up to an aortic systolic blood pressure of approximately 170 mm Hg. Stroke volume will decrease with an extreme, acute increase in aortic systolic blood pressure (Figure 10.6, excessive Ao pressure). These excessively high levels are not likely to occur in a normal person who is not exercising.

A diseased heart with depressed contractility functioning on a lower ventricular function curve (Figure 10.4) responds abnormally to an increase in afterload. The increase in end-systolic volume is larger than normal relative to the increase in end-diastolic volume and steady state stroke volume decreases (Figure 10.6). The reason for this is that the diseased myocytes respond less to stretch (increased end-diastolic volume) than normal. Ventricular steady state stroke volume decreases with increases in afterload when contractility is decreased (Figure 10.6).

Many patients with heart failure have increased peripheral vascular resistance and increased left ventricular afterload. Current treatment of this type of heart failure includes medications that reduce peripheral vascular resistance to unload the left ventricle. This type of treatment

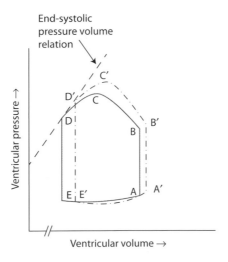

Figure 10.7 Pressure-volume loops with an increase in afterload. The broken line loop resulted after an increase in afterload.

has been shown to reduce mortality and, in some instances, results in the return of ventricular muscle structure and function toward normal.

EXAMPLES OF CHANGES IN VENTRICULAR FUNCTION

DYNAMIC EXERCISE

As the intensity of dynamic exercise, such as running, increases, cardiac sympathetic nervous activity increases. Ventricular muscle contractile state increases based on at least three simultaneous stimuli:

- Increased amounts of norepinephrine released at myocardial β receptors due to more action potentials along the cardiac sympathetic nerves (Figure 10.4, sympathetic nerves).
- More plasma epinephrine and some norepinephrine released from the adrenal medulla secondary to sympathetic stimulation of the adrenal gland (Figure 10.4, circulating catecholamines).
- A higher heart rate directly affects heart muscle function through the force-frequency relationship (Figure 10.4). This is the least important of these three factors.

Ventricular function moves to higher ventricular function curves than at rest (Figure 10.4). The end-systolic pressure-volume relation shifts leftward and is steeper (Figure 10.5). Cardiac output is greater than at rest—more blood is flowing around the body per unit time than at rest.

There are other factors to consider:

- As heart rate increases, each cardiac cycle shortens and the diastolic filling period shortens the most. With a shorter diastolic filling period there is less time for ventricular filling.
- Simultaneously, the increased amount of blood flowing around the body per minute results in more venous return to the right and left atrium per minute.
- Also, there is sympathetic stimulation of large veins like the inferior vena cava, which activates caval venous smooth muscle, reduces venous compliance, and enhances return of blood to the right atrium and ventricle. Sympathetic stimulation of myocardial cells enhances relaxation and facilitates ventricular filling. **The effects of catecholamines on heart muscle function is presented in the three-part self-study module Clinical Heart Muscle Physiology.**
- The skeletal muscle pump enhances venous return (Figure 10.1).
- Finally, during inspiration, the diaphragm moves down and increases abdominal pressure, including pressure on the inferior vena cava and its tributaries. The veins in the lower body have valves opening toward the heart, so venous blood cannot move backward. The increase in abdominal pressure pushes venous blood toward the right atrium. The increased frequency and amplitude of respiratory movements during exercise increases these effects on the veins.

The net effect of the above during exercise is variable. Measurements in humans during upright exercise show an initial rise in end-diastolic volume from rest to low level exercise, but then end-diastolic volume remains steady with further increases in exercise intensity. The steady end-diastolic volume during higher levels of upright exercise may result from the combination of less time for ventricular filling plus more blood returning per unit time. Ventricular function continues to increase at the higher levels of exercise, not due to more filling, but due to increases in ventricular contractility and heart rate.

In other words, cardiac output increases with upright endurance exercise due to an initial increase in ventricular filling and a continuing increase in heart rate and the contractile state due to increased sympathetic stimulation.

CHANGES IN POSTURE

The amount of right ventricular filling increases with lying down as venous blood becomes evenly distributed throughout the body; there is now more venous blood in the thorax than during standing. The end-diastolic volume of both ventricles increases and the ventricles move to the right on the ventricular function curve on which they are functioning. There is baro-reflex withdrawal of sympathetic stimulation of the heart and the parasympathetic nervous system becomes predominant (the carotid baroreflex is discussed in a later section Chapter 12, Circulatory Controls). The heart rate slows. Ventricular contractile state decreases, mostly due to less sympathetic stimulation of myocytes, and ventricular function moves to lower curves.

Summary: Moment-to-moment adjustments in ventricular function with, for instance, exercise or changes in posture depend on a combination of changes in the contractile state of ventricular heart muscle and the end-diastolic volume (preload).

EJECTION FRACTION

Normally, each ventricle empties until it is slightly less than half full. A normal ventricle ejects about 60% of the EDV in a beat, an ejection fraction of 0.6. Below 0.45 (some say 0.50) is considered lower than normal. The ejection fraction (EF) is a clinically important measurement and is the amount ejected by a ventricle (stroke volume; SV) relative to what was in the ventricle before ejection (end-diastolic volume; EDV).

$$EF = \frac{SV}{EDV}$$

Stroke volume is end-diastolic volume minus end-systolic volume (SV = EDV − ESV). End-systolic volume, as mentioned before, is the volume of blood in a ventricle at the end of ejection. EF can be measured non-invasively, for instance, with echocardiography.

PASSIVE (DIASTOLIC) PRESSURE-VOLUME RELATION

During diastole, the ventricle behaves like a passive compliant bag, much like a balloon. As a normal resting ventricle fills with blood, ventricular pressure increases, but to a small extent. Consider an experiment with a normal relaxed left ventricle. There are no contractions. A syringe is used to fill the left ventricle to various volumes (Figure 10.8). Left ventricular passive pressure is measured at each left ventricular passive volume. Left ventricular pressure versus left ventricular volume is plotted (Figure 10.8). Again, note that this is in a noncontracting, relaxed heart. Why does the pressure go up with an increase in volume of the noncontracting left ventricle?

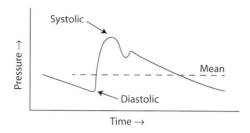

Figure 11.1 Aortic pulse and mean blood pressure. Mean arterial blood pressure is discussed in the text. Diastolic blood pressure here refers to pressure in the aorta, not in the left ventricle. Aortic systolic blood pressure is measured at the peak of pressure development.

transiently exceed peripheral runoff and aortic volume and mean aortic pressure will increase. As you would expect with a siphon, increased mean arterial pressure results in increased runoff. A new steady state is attained with a higher cardiac output, a higher mean aortic pressure, and more runoff. For a given increase in cardiac output, the amount of increase of the mean aortic pressure depends on aortic stiffness.

AORTIC STIFFNESS

As noted above, when the aortic wall is stiff a given increase in aortic volume will result in a bigger increase in mean aortic pressure than when the wall of the aorta is less stiff. Stiffness can be measured in an aortic segment, such as might be obtained at autopsy (Figure 11.2).

In Figure 11.2, a segment of aorta was removed at autopsy from various age people. Each aortic segment was attached at one end to a syringe and at the other to a pressure gauge (Figure 11.2). Then each aortic segment was filled to various volumes with saline. The resulting pressure inside the aortic segment at each volume was plotted against the volume (Figure 11.2).

In this experiment, external pressure, P_e, is atmospheric and remains constant. Inside pressure (P_i) increased as saline was injected and transmural pressure (P_t) ($P_t = P_i - P_e$) increased.

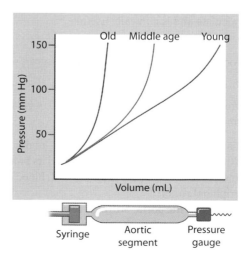

Figure 11.2 Pressure-volume relation in aortic segments from young, middle age, and old people.

P_t increases because, as vessel radius increases in response to fluid injection, circumference increases. The connective tissue fibers in the vessel wall are stretched, wall force increases, and pressure inside (P_i) rises. The vertical axis, pressure, is P_i (Figure 11.2).

Stiffness of the aorta and other large blood vessels vary with, for example, age. Less volume is needed in the aorta of an old person to reach, for example, a pressure of 90 mm Hg than for someone who is middle age or young (Figure 11.2). This means the aorta is less distensible, less compliant or stiffer in the old person than in the younger person. The explanation is that connective tissue gets stiffer with age. Also note throughout the physiologic mean pressure range (approximately 70–105 mm Hg) the relationship of pressure with volume is close to linear in younger people and becomes more steeply upsloping with increasing age. This again is a manifestation of the normal aorta getting stiffer with age.

At a given cardiac output and peripheral runoff, the steady state blood volume and stretch of the aorta in an older person might result in a higher aortic blood pressure, particularly systolic blood pressure than in a younger person. Why systolic? Because aortic volume is maximal at peak systolic blood pressure.

RELATIONSHIP OF PRESSURE, FLOW, AND RESISTANCE

$$Q = \frac{\bar{P}_1 - \bar{P}_2}{R}$$

Q is blood flow per unit time and R is vascular resistance. In the overall systemic circulation Q is the same as cardiac output (CO), $\bar{P}_1$ is mean aortic blood pressure, and $\bar{P}_2$ is mean right atrial blood pressure. In the pulmonary circulation, the pressures of interest would be the mean pulmonary artery blood pressure and the mean left atrial blood pressure.

Resistance in the systemic circulation resides mostly in the arterioles and is discussed below. Resistance influences peripheral runoff. High resistance impedes runoff and low resistance results in an increase in runoff. Below there is a discussion of why changes in runoff due to changes in resistance can be transient.

DETERMINANTS OF PULSE PRESSURE

The aorta and its branches constitute a confined system with the aortic valve at its proximal end and peripheral vascular resistance and peripheral runoff at the other end. The left ventricular ejection of blood into the aorta is rapid during the initial part of ejection. This initial rapid left ventricular ejection exceeds peripheral runoff. Therefore, aortic volume increases, the aortic wall is stretched, and aortic blood pressure increases to the peak aortic pressure, the aortic systolic pressure.

Aortic pressure falls after the peak because:

- Left ventricular myocardial relaxation becomes more manifest, slowing the rate of ejection of blood into the aorta. There is no further release of Ca^{2+} from the terminal cisternae in ventricular myocytes and Ca^{2+} uptake by the longitudinal portion of the sarcoplasmic reticulum is proceeding. **Activation of contraction and relaxation are presented in detail in the three-part self-study module Clinical Heart Muscle Physiology**.
- Peripheral runoff begins to exceed the amount of blood ejected by the left ventricle and aortic volume begins to fall. Aortic pressure falls as aortic volume decreases (Figure 11.2).

As you know from the earlier section on the cardiac cycle (Chapter 9, Cardiac Cycle, Heart Sounds and Murmurs), at the end of ejection the left ventricle is not able to sustain forward flow because of the extant of myocardial relaxation. The column of blood in the aortic root momentarily moves backward toward the aortic valve and the valve closes. Once the aortic valve closes the aorta is then sealed at its ventricular end. But at the other end of the arterial system peripheral runoff continues. Blood exits from the arterial system into the capillary bed through the arterioles and aortic blood pressure falls. The fall in aortic blood pressure continues until the next cardiac cycle results in aortic valve opening and ventricular ejection. The lowest level the aortic blood pressure gets to, at the instant before the aortic valve opens, is the aortic diastolic blood pressure (Figure 11.3, point 2 and Figure 11.1).

The increase of aortic blood pressure after the aortic valve opens results from early rapid left ventricular ejection. About 80% of the stroke volume is ejected during early rapid ejection. The blood pressure increase starts from the aortic diastolic blood pressure level when the aortic valve opens and reaches the peak aortic and ventricular systolic level. This rise from diastolic to peak systolic blood pressure is the pulse pressure, as described above.

From the above it should be obvious that the peak aortic systolic pressure is strongly dependent on stroke volume. Also, the aortic diastolic blood pressure is directly dependent on the amount of peripheral runoff. Since peripheral vascular resistance is a major determinant of the amount of peripheral runoff, peripheral vascular resistance also strongly influences the level of aortic diastolic blood pressure.

Finally, for any given amount of stroke volume, pulse pressure will be greater the stiffer the aorta. This corresponds to what is stated above about aortic stiffness. A given volume increment added to a stiffer aorta will result in a greater pressure increase than in a less stiff aorta (Figure 11.2).

Note: The thrust of blood into the aorta from the left ventricle during ejection generates a pressure wave that starts from the aortic root and travels throughout the arterial system. The pressure wave can be palpated peripherally, for instance, over the radial artery at the wrist.

All the above comments also apply to the right ventricle and pulmonary artery, but the blood pressure levels are much lower due to the very low pulmonary vascular resistance and relatively compliant (low stiffness) pulmonary artery wall.

EXAMPLES OF PULSE PRESSURE CHANGES

With a slow heart rate, there is a longer time for peripheral runoff between heartbeats. With more time for peripheral runoff more blood can leave the aorta and aortic diastolic blood pressure decreases. The slower heart rate also results in more time for ventricular filling and an increase in end-diastolic volume, and stroke volume increases. The rise in stroke volume increases systolic blood pressure. There is then a tendency for a larger pulse pressure when heart rate is slow. Mean pressure may not significantly change. For instance, say that peak aortic systolic blood pressure before a decrease in heart rate is 122 mm Hg and diastolic is 80 mm Hg. The mean blood pressure is $80 + (42/3) = 94$ mm Hg. After the increase in heart rate the values might be 133/70 mm Hg with a mean of $70 + (63/3) = 91$ mm Hg. The mean arterial pressure does not significantly change in this example.

Consider another simplified example. Aortic systolic, pulse, and mean blood pressures increase with an increase in stroke volume. An increase in stroke volume as an isolated event is not likely, but this simplified scenario is useful as a learning tool. In this example neither heart rate nor peripheral vascular resistance change. An increase in mean arterial blood pressure will increase steady state peripheral runoff. The increase in peripheral runoff in combination with

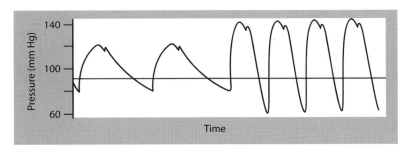

Figure 11.3 Aortic blood pressure changes with dynamic exercise. The horizontal line represents mean blood pressure at 93 mm Hg.

the increase in stroke volume and aortic systolic blood pressure at a constant heart rate result in almost no change in the aortic diastolic pressure. With no change in heart rate the time available for runoff is unchanged. The aorta starts from a higher volume and systolic pressure, but there is no increase in time for runoff and the diastolic pressure is slightly greater or unchanged.

Figure 11.3 illustrates another change in pulse pressure. In this case, stroke volume and heart rate increase whereas peripheral vascular resistance (another term for this is systemic vascular resistance) decreases. Aortic systolic blood pressure increases and aortic diastolic blood pressure decreases, but without a change in mean blood pressure. This latter response occurs in, for instance, upright dynamic exercise, such as jogging on a treadmill, and is analyzed in detail in Figure 11.4. Heart rate and stroke volume increase due to increased sympathetic nerve activity to the heart. The heart rate increase is also related to decreased parasympathetic nerve activity to the sinoatrial node. The decrease in peripheral vascular resistance is primarily the result of arteriolar vasodilatation in working skeletal muscles, an effect of local metabolic control, which is discussed later (Chapter 12, Circulatory Controls).

The next example is what occurs with an increase in peripheral vascular resistance (Figure 11.5). The initial response to an increase in peripheral vascular resistance is a decrease in peripheral runoff and an increase in aortic volume, stiffness, and diastolic and mean blood pressures (Figure 11.5). Since the circulation behaves as a siphon, the increase in mean aortic blood pressure brings peripheral runoff back toward what it originally was. The increase in aortic stiffness (Figure 11.5) refers to the increase in aortic volume causing a shift onto a steeper portion of an aortic pressure, volume relation (Figure 11.2). Aortic systolic blood pressure also increases. Left ventricular stroke volume (not mentioned in Figure 11.5) is little affected by the increased left ventricular afterload, which is explained in Chapter 10, Ventricular Function, Afterload.

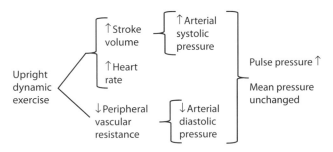

Figure 11.4 Factors that result in an aortic pulse pressure increase and a stable aortic mean blood pressure with dynamic exercise.

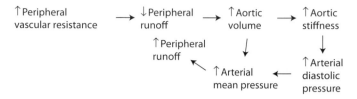

↑ Peripheral vascular resistance → ↓ Peripheral runoff → ↑ Aortic volume → ↑ Aortic stiffness

↑ Peripheral runoff

↑ Arterial mean pressure ← ↑ Arterial diastolic pressure

Figure 11.5 Responses to an increase in peripheral vascular resistance.

RESISTANCE

The following formula relating pressure, flow, and resistance was discussed earlier:

$$Q = \frac{\bar{P}_1 - \bar{P}_2}{R}$$

By rearranging this formula, resistance to liquid flowing in a tube can be defined by the following ratio:

$$\text{Resistance to Flow (R)} = \frac{\text{Pressure Drop from Point 1 to 2}}{\text{Total Flow from Point 1 to 2}} = \frac{\bar{P}_1 - \bar{P}_2}{Q}$$

There are several factors that influence resistance, including the cross-sectional area of the tube, the length of the tube (L), and the viscosity (η) of the fluid flowing in the tube.

$$R = \frac{8\eta L}{\pi r^4}$$

The radius, r, π and 8 appear as part of the mathematical derivation. Substitution of the formula for R into the first equation results in a relationship called Poiseuille's law. Poiseuille, a French physician and physicist, made empirical observations of fluid flow in tubes that eventually were related mathematically to Newton's observations and calculations regarding laminar flow.

POISEUILLE'S LAW

$$Q = \frac{\pi(\bar{P}_1 - \bar{P}_2)r^4}{8\eta L}$$

where
- Q = Flow rate in volume/unit time
- r = Blood vessel radius
- $\bar{P}_1$ = Mean pressure of the fluid upstream from the location in the blood vessel where this law is being applied
- $\bar{P}_2$ = Downstream mean pressure
- L = Length of blood vessel between the two points where the pressures are measured
- η = Viscosity
- $\frac{\pi}{8}$ = Constant related to integrating flow over the total cross-section of a blood vessel

VARIABLES IN POISEUILLE'S LAW

- η: It is hardly surprising that η, viscosity, is in the denominator. The "stickier" or "thicker" a fluid, the slower it will flow in response to a given pressure difference; for instance, flow of ketchup versus wine.

  Red blood cells (RBCs) make up a large part of blood volume and the viscosity of blood is strongly dependent on the RBC content of blood. Normally, RBCs make up about 40% of the volume of blood and the viscosity of blood, its internal viscosity, is about 4 times that of water. The rubbing and bumping of RBCs is the main contributor to the internal viscous forces of blood. If the number of RBCs increases, viscosity increases. In anemia, viscosity is less than normal and that is one reason why Q is greater than normal in anemia (and why murmurs may occur—see the earlier discussion of turbulence in Chapter 8, How the Circulation Works).

  The viscosity of blood also depends to some degree on the velocity of blood flow. At extremely low flow rates blood cells tend to stack up in columns and rub more against each other, and apparent viscosity is greater than at high flow rates. This type of "sludging" is important to consider when someone is in shock due to low blood flow. At higher flow rates blood cells tend to migrate to the center of the moving column of blood where energy and velocity is greatest, but they are randomly distributed within that center region. This leaves a "lubricating" layer of cell-free plasma near the vessel wall, and viscosity is less than at lower flow rates.

- $(\bar{P}_1 - \bar{P}_2)$: Pressure potential energy generated by myocardial work. Discussed previously in Chapter 8, How the Circulation Works.

- r^4: The radius (r) is of critical importance. Note that flow varies directly with the fourth power of the radius. With blood vessel obstruction, without other changes, flow will decrease relative to the fourth power of the decrease in the radius. If blood vessel radius decreases by 1/2, blood flow will decrease 16-fold, assuming other variables do not change.

- L: L, vessel length, does not acutely change. The exception to this is the stretch of lung intra-alveolar blood vessels during deep inspiration.

REGIONAL CHARACTERISTICS OF ARTERIAL BLOOD PRESSURE

The mean pressure in the aorta and its major branches is much higher than in the capillary bed (Figure 11.6). A steep pressure decrease occurs in the region of the circulation made up of small muscular arteries with a diameter <100 μm and arterioles (Figure 11.6). The fall in mean pressure is particularly steep starting with an arteriolar diameter of 50 μm. The location of the sharp fall in mean blood pressure indicates the site of most resistance in the systemic circulation—the small muscular arteries and arterioles.

Arterioles are characterized by a large ratio of muscular wall thickness to the small lumen diameter. Contraction or relaxation of arteriolar smooth muscle results in changes in arteriolar lumen radius and, therefore, in resistance. Arterioles are innervated by autonomic nerves in some organs, are sensitive to interstitial chemical changes in some organs, or have smooth muscle myocytes that are stretch-activated in some organs. Combinations of these controlling influences are discussed below in a section on circulatory controls (Chapter 12, Criculatory Controls). Parasympathetic nerve action potentials induce vasodilation in a few organs, for instance, the surface blood vessels of the brain. Elsewhere they have limited effects on controlling blood flow.

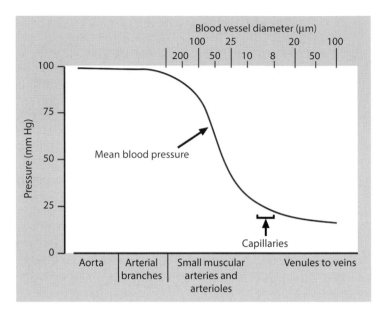

Figure 11.6 Mean blood pressure at locations in the circulation.

SERIES VASCULAR RESISTANCE

Arterioles are the major resistance vessel in the systemic circulation and there are arterioles in every organ. In some organs, the kidney and the gut for instance, there is more than one set of arterioles and in these organs the resistances are in series. Resistances (R) in series are additive:

$$R_t = R_1 + R_2 + R_3 + \cdots$$

R_t is total resistance and is illustrated in Figure 11.7c.

PARALLEL VASCULAR RESISTANCE

The reciprocal of resistances in parallel are additive.

$$(1/R_t) = (1/R_1) + (1/R_2) + \cdots$$

Notice that the more resistances added in parallel, the less the total resistance, R_t. This may seem counterintuitive at first. Each blood vessel added does have resistance, but it also adds another conduit for fluid flow (Figure 11.7b). Most organs are parallel to each other in the peripheral circulation. Adding resistances R_2 and R_3 in parallel with R_1 in Figure 11.7b adds multiple parallel paths, reduces total resistance, and increases flow.

VASCULAR CONDUCTANCE

The reciprocal of resistance is conductance, $C = (1/R)$. Series resistances are additive as noted above, $R_t = R_1 + R_2 + R_3$, and conductance equals $1/R_t$. The more the series resistance the

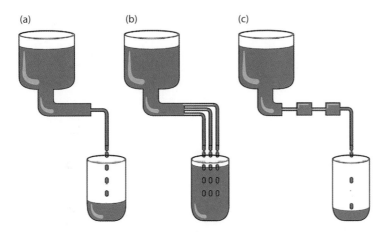

Figure 11.7 Resistances. Single resistance in **(a)**, three parallel resistances in **(b)**, and two series resistances in **(c)**. The volume in each bottom container accumulates over the same amount of time; flow rate is greatest in **b**, least in **c**, and intermediate in **a**.

greater the value for R_t and the lower the conductance. Compare the fluid flow in c with a in Figure 11.7. The reciprocals of parallel resistances are additive and the more the number of parallel resistances, the lower the overall resistance, R_t. As R_t falls, conductance increases. Compare the fluid flow in b with a in Figure 11.7.

IN VIVO RESISTANCES

The branches of the aorta are parallel to each other. Compare, for instance, the renal arteries with the arteries to the extremities and the gastrointestinal tract. With this parallel arrangement vasoconstriction and reduced blood flow (conductance) in one organ can occur with minimal effects on total resistance or systemic blood flow. What often happens is that increased resistance and reduced blood flow in one organ can be accompanied by reduced resistance and increased blood flow elsewhere. For instance, in upright dynamic exercise, such as on a stationary bicycle, blood flow to skeletal muscles and the heart increases while it decreases to the gut and kidney.

BLOOD VOLUME DISTRIBUTION

Distribution of blood volume as well as sites of resistance is a function of the geometry and structure of the circulation. In a resting person, approximately 2/3 of the circulating blood is in the venous side of the circulation. The veins are thin-walled with a modest amount of smooth muscle and easily expand. They are well suited to accommodate a large volume of blood. The venous portion of the peripheral circulation is characterized by high volume and low pressure.

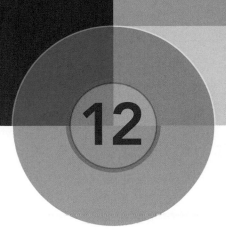

Circulatory controls

INTRODUCTION

There are multiple levels of control operating simultaneously in the circulation. It is not unusual in biological systems to have multiple control mechanisms acting to maintain an internal steady state. The discussion here treats each control system individually, but keep in mind they all operate together to harmonize cardiovascular function to maintain a normal internal environment.

Rapid control of blood pressure is accomplished in large part by baroreceptors and the central nervous system reflexes they are part of. Another term for baroreceptor is "pressure receptor" or pressoreceptor. The efferent part of this reflex system occurs over sympathetic and parasympathetic nerves. These neural reflexes are essential for rapid responses to changes in blood pressure. Neural reflexes quickly stabilize blood pressure levels that are dependent over the long term on blood volume. Blood volume is strongly influenced by hormonal control of salt and water excretion, another type of circulatory control. Hormonal control of salt and water excretion is a slower type of baroreflex control system and also responds to changes in blood osmolality.

ARTERIAL NEURAL BARORECEPTORS

The major neural baroreceptors are the carotid sinuses bilaterally and the aortic arch.

STRUCTURE

CAROTID SINUS

The carotid sinus is located at the junction of the internal and common carotid arteries (Figure 12.1). There are two key features of the carotid sinus wall that make the sinus a good blood pressure sensor. The wall is very distensible (highly compliant) and there is an extensively branched matrix of stretch-activated nerve endings embedded in the wall. Action potentials generated by stretch of the nerve matrix travel along the carotid sinus nerves bilaterally to the medulla oblongata. The medulla contains integrating centers.

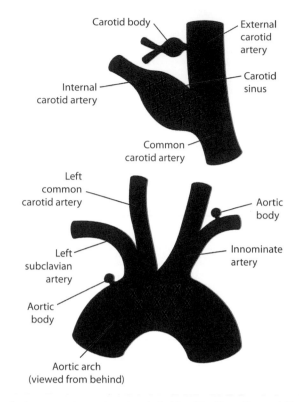

Figure 12.1 Two major baroreceptor regions located at the X's. (From Barrett KE et al. *Ganong's Review of Medical Physiology*, 23rd ed. New York, NY: McGraw-Hill; 2010. With permission of McGraw-Hill.)

AORTIC ARCH

A matrix of stretch-activated nerve endings is embedded in the wall of the aortic arch, like that in the carotid sinus (Figure 12.1). The function of the two arterial baroreceptor areas is similar. The carotid sinus baroreceptor has been more thoroughly studied and will be discussed here.

FUNCTION OF THE CAROTID SINUS BARORECEPTOR

CLINICAL CASE

A clinical case emphasizes the importance of understanding neural baroreceptor function:

A 77-year-old man recently began treatment with beta₁ blocking and vasodilating drugs for heart failure. In the last few days he has had increasing difficulty with dizziness and blurred vision when changing posture from lying or sitting to standing upright. These symptoms are worse when first standing in the morning. His blood pressure while sitting is 118/72 mm Hg and after standing, resting for less than 3 minutes his blood pressure is 92/60 mm Hg. A decrease in systolic blood pressure within 3 minutes of changing from sitting to standing is normally <20 mm Hg systolic and <10 mm Hg diastolic.

What is the physiological basis of this problem and how should it be treated? The answers are dependent on an understanding of the neural baroreflex.

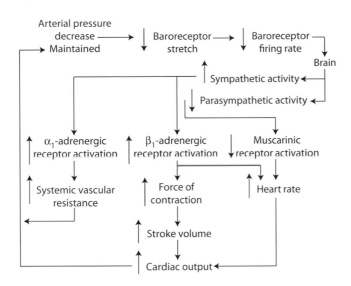

Figure 12.2 Flow diagram of the response of the carotid sinus baroreceptor reflex to a decrease in arterial blood pressure. The flow starts at the upper right with an "arterial pressure decrease" and the negative feedback loop concludes back at the upper right with arterial pressure increased to maintain a blood pressure adequate for organ function.

An arterial blood pressure decrease (Figure 12.2, arterial pressure decrease) results in less expansion of the carotid sinus and less stretch of its wall (↓ baroreceptor stretch) and the embedded nerves. Less stretch of the nerves results in less action potentials (↓ baroreceptor firing rate) along the carotid sinus afferent nerves to cardiovascular centers in the medulla. Medullary centers in the brain integrate this incoming information and the result is more action potentials along sympathetic and less along parasympathetic nerves (Figure 12.2).

Less stretch of the carotid sinus leads to more sympathetic nerve activity—potentially confusing until you consider the following. All the cardiovascular control systems are operating all the time. They do not turn on when needed and then turn off. The carotid sinus wall is always stretched by arterial blood pressure and there are continuous carotid sinus nerve action potentials, the frequency of which increase with more stretch of the sinus and decrease with less stretch. Carotid sinus nerve action potentials act to inhibit the sympathetic nerve output from the medullary cardiovascular centers. When blood pressure falls and there is less stretch of the carotid sinus wall and less carotid sinus nerve action potentials to the medulla there is less suppression of the sympathetic nerve output and increased action potentials in the sympathetic nerves to the heart and blood vessels. The converse is true of the parasympathetic system. Basal carotid sinus nerve activity maintains activation of parasympathetic nerve cell bodies in the medulla and reduced carotid sinus nerve activity results in less activation and less parasympathetic nerve activity.

The result of more sympathetic activity and less parasympathetic activity is illustrated in Figure 12.2. Start at the upper left of Figure 12.2 with a decrease in arterial blood pressure. A common example of a normal decrease in arterial blood pressure is a change of posture from lying to standing. The effects of gravity result in a significant shift of venous blood to the lower body with standing, estimated at 800–1000 mL. The venous volume shift substantially reduces thoracic blood volume (Figure 12.3). The right atrium and ventricle fill less (decreased right atrial mean pressure in Figure 12.3) and stroke volume decreases (Figure 12.3) (this is a

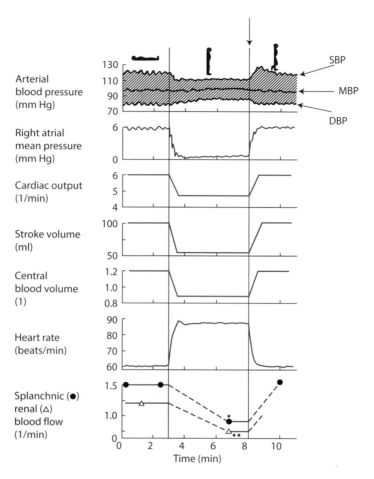

Figure 12.3 Hemodynamic effects of posture change and the skeletal muscle pump. SBP is systolic arterial blood pressure, DBP is diastolic arterial blood pressure, and MBP is mean arterial blood pressure. The figures at the top indicate a transition from supine to standing and then standing with leg contractions. Other details are discussed in the text. (From Rowell LB. *Human Circulation Regulation during Physical Stress*, 1986, by permission of Oxford University Press.)

good time to review the earlier material on Frank–Starling law of the heart). After a few heartbeats, the same happens in the left atrium and ventricle. Reduced left ventricular stroke volume results in a decrease in arterial systolic pressure (SBP in Figure 12.3 with standing) and less stretch of the carotid sinus (Figure 12.2). The result is a decrease in action potential generation in the carotid sinus nerve endings with a decrease in action potential frequency over those nerves to the brain (Figure 12.2). Figure 12.2 outlines the reflex loop.

Note that the reflex loops act to maintain mean arterial blood pressure (MBP in Figure 12.3). Normal resting standing arterial systolic blood pressure is less than what it was when lying down due to the reduced stroke volume (Figure 12.3) and arterial diastolic blood pressure is increased (DBP in Figure 12.3) due to peripheral vasoconstriction. The peripheral vasoconstriction is a result of more sympathetic activity to peripheral arteriolar smooth muscle alpha receptors (Figure 12.2). Reduced splanchnic and renal blood flow (Figure 12.3) is a result of the vasoconstriction.

As noted above, the carotid (and aortic) baroreceptor is a rapid, nervous, millisecond response control system. One cannot stand up and remain upright free of symptoms unless this rapid response system works properly. The carotid baroreceptor compensates for the effects of gravity on the cardiovascular system, but gravity does not go away. All the time one is standing gravity acts to shift venous blood to the lower body. There is increased sympathetic input to venous alpha receptors that stiffens the wall of the veins and helps to move venous blood toward the right atrium, but a reduced ventricular end-diastolic volume and stroke volume persist all the time one is standing as compared with lying down or sitting. Central blood volume remains reduced during standing as compared with lying down despite the stiffening of the veins (Figure 12.3).

Figure 12.3 also nicely illustrates the effects of the skeletal muscle pump during standing. At the 8-minute time mark (top arrow, right vertical line) the upright individual began contracting and relaxing leg muscles without walking. As described before, contraction of leg muscles squeezes the deep veins between muscle bundles. These veins have valves. Venous blood is pushed toward the heart with leg muscle contraction and cannot flow back when the valves close with leg muscle relaxation. The repeated cycle of contraction and relaxation pumps blood toward the heart. Note the return of all the parameters back to the levels when the individual was lying supine. This would be a good time to revisit earlier notes on ventricular function and the Frank–Starling law of the heart where the skeletal muscle pump is also discussed.

CLINICAL CASE REVISITED

As you will recall, the 77-year-old man recently began treatment with beta₁ blocking and vasodilating drugs for heart failure and he is now having difficulty with dizziness and blurred vision when changing posture from lying or sitting to standing upright. His blood pressure decreases more than normal with changing posture from sitting to standing. The blood pressure decrease is enough to limit brain blood flow. I hope it is obvious the beta₁ blocking and vasodilating drugs are interfering excessively with the patient's neural baroreflex response. The medications are appropriate for heart failure therapy, but the doses or drugs will have to be changed to reduce the patient's problem with postural low arterial blood pressure or orthostatic hypotension.

If for some reason arterial blood pressure increases and remains chronically elevated, such as in the disease "high blood pressure (hypertension)," the baroreceptors adapt and control blood pressure at the new higher level.

HORMONAL CONTROLS

RENIN-ANGIOTENSIN-ALDOSTERONE SYSTEM (RAAS)

RAAS is involved in slower, longer term control of blood pressure than the neural baroreceptor system, but both act together to maintain steady state blood pressure levels. A major feature of RAAS is the control of extracellular fluid volume and thereby the long-term control of vascular volume and arterial blood pressure. **There is a detailed presentation of RAAS, including animated illustrations, in the self-study module the Pathophysiology of Hypovolemic Shock**.

e

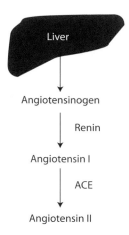

Figure 12.5 Actions of renin and angiotensin converting enzyme (ACE).

ANTIDIURETIC HORMONE (ADH) OR VASOPRESSIN

ADH is synthesized in the hypothalamus and then diffuses along neuronal axons in the pituitary stalk to where it is stored in and available for release from the posterior pituitary gland. The primary stimulus for release of ADH from the posterior pituitary is an increase in plasma osmolality. In dehydration, for instance, plasma osmolality increases; this is sensed by hypothalamic osmoreceptors and ADH release increases. ADH release from the posterior pituitary gland also increases in response to a large decrease in blood volume, such as in hemorrhage. **This is presented in the self-study module The Pathophysiology of Hypovolemic Shock.**

ADH has two major actions. It acts on the kidneys to increase water reabsorption in the distal tubule. This is its major action in normal people. If there is a large enough decrease in circulating blood volume, such as in hemorrhage, enough ADH may be released so that blood levels are high enough to result in vasoconstriction. Hence the name "vasopressin." **This is discussed further in the self-study module The Pathophysiology of Hypovolemic Shock.**

ATRIAL AND BRAIN NATRIURETIC PEPTIDES

Atrial natriuretic peptide (ANP) is produced by atrial cells. Brain natriuretic peptide (BNP) is produced by ventricular cells. BNP was first discovered in pig brain tissue, hence the name. Subsequently, the primary source was found to be from cardiac ventricular myocardium. BNP is also produced by the atria, but in smaller amounts than in the ventricles because of the smaller atrial muscle mass. ANP and BNP are released into the blood and act as hormones. C-type natriuretic peptide (CNP) is produced in endothelial cells and mostly acts locally in a paracrine or autocrine manner on vascular smooth muscle.

Release of ANP and BNP into the bloodstream is triggered by increases in atrial and ventricular wall tension due either to chamber distention or increased chamber pressure or a combination of both. The hormonal actions of ANP and BNP can be divided into those that occur in a normal person and actions that become important in, for instance, heart disease.

Consider, for example, a change in posture in a normal person from standing to lying. There is a redistribution of venous blood volume so that atrial and ventricular filling increase and wall tension increases. More ANP and BNP are produced and secreted into the bloodstream. They relax vascular smooth muscle and result in peripheral arteriolar vasodilation, which modulates the rise in arterial blood pressure related to increased left ventricular stroke volume with lying down. ANP and BNP also decrease kidney reabsorption of Na^+ resulting in more Na^+ and water excretion. The change in posture from standing to lying increases atrial and ventricular filling and ANP and BNP natriuresis acts to reduce plasma volume and atrial and ventricular filling. This is another example of negative feedback circulatory control. ANP and BNP also inhibit renin secretion and aldosterone production, an effect that also will relax arterioles and enhance kidney salt and water excretion.

The actions of ANP and BNP become important in, for example, heart disease. For example, increased left ventricular pressure and wall tension in aortic valvular stenosis results in left ventricular hypertrophy and a stiffer chamber with increased filling pressures. The increased filling pressures result in an increase in left atrial pressure and wall tension. More than normal amounts of ANF and BNF are produced and released into the bloodstream.

Patients with aortic valvular stenosis and left ventricular hypertrophy eventually develop heart failure that is characterized by myocardial and vascular remodeling, and myocardial apoptosis and fibrosis. Relatively recent findings show that ANP and BNP act to reduce these adverse myocardial and vascular changes in heart failure. The clinical use of these beneficial effects of ANP and BNP is currently being investigated. The action of natriuretic peptides, particularly ANP, is terminated by enzymatic degradation by neprilysin. Neprilysin is produced in vascular endothelial cells and the tubular cells of the kidney. Clinical testing of neprilysin inhibitors have been carried out recently and show promise for heart failure treatment.

In addition to their physiologic actions, ANP and BNP blood level increases have diagnostic and prognostic significance. Increased blood levels of the natriuretic peptides are diagnostic of hemodynamic overload, ventricular dysfunction, and heart failure. Blood levels of these peptides are used to assess prognosis and to monitor therapy.

CNP primarily acts in a paracrine and autocrine manner and has little hormonal and natriuretic action, but is still classified as a natriuretic peptide.

VASCULAR ENDOTHELIAL FACTORS

The endothelial cell lining of the vasculature previously was thought to be a single cell layer functioning only as a smooth liner and passive filter. This is now known to be incorrect. Endothelial cells are metabolically active and produce vasoactive substances that act mostly as paracrine hormones. These vasoactive substances are produced by the endothelial cells and diffuse through the vessel wall to act on the local vascular smooth muscle. Endothelial cell vasoactive substances act locally to relax vascular smooth muscle in normal arterial resistance vessels. They also prevent clotting (Figure 12.6).

NO

Nitric oxide (NO) plays a prominent role in vasodilation of larger arterial resistance vessels and in veins. NO acts through cGMP to decrease smooth muscle cytosolic Ca^{2+} and relax local vascular smooth muscle (Figure 12.6). There is continual, basal release of NO from endothelial cells stimulated by the continual shear stress of blood flow. Once released it is quickly inactivated and its continuing action depends on continual release. Blood flow rubbing on the

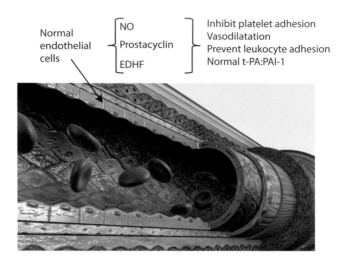

Normal endothelial cells
- NO
- Prostacyclin
- EDHF

Inhibit platelet adhesion
Vasodilatation
Prevent leukocyte adhesion
Normal t-PA:PAI-1

Figure 12.6 Endothelial cell factors produced in and released from normal endothelial cells.

luminal surface of endothelial cells (shear forces) stimulates them to produce and release NO. NO production and release increase when flow into resistance vessels increases. Thus, more blood flow is accommodated by vasodilation to match vessel lumen size with flow. Venous endothelial cells also produce NO.

Production and release of NO is also stimulated by products of clotting such as thrombin, serotonin, and ADP produced by aggregating platelets, and other chemicals such as bradykinin and histamine. NO, in turn, inhibits the clotting cascade and reduces the likelihood of completed clot formation and lumen obstruction (Figure 12.6).

NO production and release is stimulated by acetylcholine. Parasympathetic nerves are found in the outer layers of blood vessel walls, but some acetylcholine can diffuse through the wall and affect the endothelium.

PROSTACYCLIN

Prostacyclin is also released in arterial resistance vessels by shear stress related to blood flow. It relaxes local vascular smooth muscle and prevents clotting. Prostacyclin analogues are used clinically to relax pulmonary vascular smooth muscle in patients with abnormally high pulmonary vascular resistance and elevated pulmonary artery blood pressure (a clinical condition known as pulmonary hypertension).

ENDOTHELIUM-DERIVED HYPERPOLARIZING FACTORS (EDHF)

EDHF opens smooth muscle sarcolemma Ca^{2+}-activated K^+ channels. This makes it easier for K^+ to leave the smooth muscle cells. The smooth muscle cells become hyperpolarized and less likely to depolarize and contract. EDHF secretion is increased by shear forces, but it also mediates the vasodilatory effects of bradykinin on vascular smooth muscle. There are several EDHFs and one is hydrogen peroxide. EDHF seems to play a bigger role in the smaller arterioles whereas NO is more important in the small muscular arteries and larger arterioles.

EFFECTS ON BLOOD CLOTTING

Endothelial cells produce and release tissue plasminogen activator (t-PA) and plasminogen-activator inhibitor type 1 (PAI-1) (Figure 12.5). A normal ratio is important for normal fibrinolysis to prevent inappropriate clot formation.

DYSFUNCTIONAL ENDOTHELIUM

Reduced production and release of NO is characteristic of dysfunctional endothelium (Figure 12.7). Less NO release from endothelial cells tips the balance of endothelial control toward vascular smooth muscle contraction and clot formation. Abnormalities of endothelial function can be found in, for instance, the endothelium overlying atherosclerotic plaques and in hypercholesterolemia in the absence of discrete atheroma and obstruction. Changes in endothelial cell function are proving to be important in the pathogenesis of atherosclerotic coronary and cerebral vascular disease and in heart failure.

ENDOTHELINS

There are several endothelin isoforms produced by vascular endothelial cells and other tissues. Interaction of endothelin with receptors on vascular smooth muscle results in sustained contraction. Its synthesis and release is induced by several stimuli including angiotensin II, norepinephrine, and inflammatory cytokines, and it plays a role in the generalized vasoconstriction in some pathological states, such as heart failure. Endothelins play a much smaller role in normal resistance vessels other than to contribute to vessel tone.

One of the endothelin isoforms interacts with receptors on endothelial cells. It is produced by endothelial cells and affects local endothelial cell function. This isoform enhances NO production and favors vasodilation. So endothelin actions can favor vasoconstriction and vasodilation—this is a good example of dual competitive actions that are not uncommon in

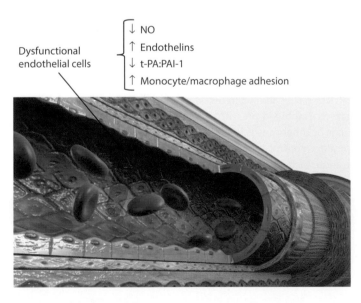

Dysfunctional endothelial cells

↓ NO
↑ Endothelins
↓ t-PA:PAI-1
↑ Monocyte/macrophage adhesion

Figure 12.7 Abnormal endothelial cell function.

circulatory control. Which wins out, vascular smooth muscle relaxation or contraction? That depends on the net effect of multiple factors. For instance, the combination of an excessive increase in circulating catecholamines and angiotensin II and increased release of endothelin from vascular endothelial cells (Figure 12.7) in heart failure results in vasoconstriction.

THROMBOXANE

Thromboxane is produced primarily by platelet aggregation. Vascular endothelial cell damage, for instance, in the region of an atherosclerotic plaque can result in changes in endothelial cell function that attract blood platelets and induce them to produce thromboxane, a potent vasoconstrictor. As noted above, abnormal endothelial cells overlying an atherosclerotic plaque produce less vasodilators, such as nitric oxide and prostacyclins, relative to endothelin. The tendency toward vasoconstriction increases the obstruction produced by the plaque and further reduces blood flow and organ blood supply.

Thromboxane can play a role in the vasoconstriction associated with such pathologic states as atherosclerosis, pulmonary hypertension, heart failure, and kidney failure.

CLOTTING

Abnormal endothelial cells produce a lower t-PA:PAI-1 ratio (Figure 12.7). There is less blood fibrinolytic activity and a greater tendency toward thrombosis.

CHEMORECEPTORS

It is doubtful whether the normal circulation is under any influence of chemoreceptors. Chemoreceptors do play a key role in regulation of normal respiration.

Chemoreceptor control of the circulation can become important in some abnormalities. For instance, with severe enough hemorrhage to result in a major drop in blood pressure, blood flow decreases in chemoreceptors, for instance, in the aortic and carotid bodies* (Figure 12.1). PO_2 and pH then decrease and PCO_2 increases in chemoreceptor interstitial tissue. These local changes in the chemoreceptor interstitium generate more action potentials over afferent nerves from the chemoreceptor to medullary vasoconstrictor centers. Increased sympathetic outflow from the vasoconstrictor centers to α-receptors around the body then contributes to the generalized vasoconstriction that characterizes severe hemorrhage. This is a body survival mechanism to maintain central blood pressure and blood flow to the brain and heart in the face of severe hemorrhage or other causes of a major abnormal drop in blood pressure.

Central respiratory control centers are also affected in the above scenario. Increased frequency of respiration, tachypnea, accompanies severe hemorrhage.

LOCAL METABOLIC CONTROL

Most organs have local metabolic control of blood flow. An increase in organ work and metabolism results in changes in the organ's interstitium that causes arteriolar

---

* Do not confuse the carotid *bodies*, chemoreceptor organs, with the carotid *sinus* baroreceptors (Figure 14.1).

vasodilatation. Increased organ work and metabolism results in the following changes in the interstitium:

- ↑ Adenosine
- ↑ K^+
- ↑ Lactic acid
- ↓ PO_2 (more O_2 taken up by the organ cells)
- ↑ PCO_2
- ↓ pH (↑CO_2 plus interstitial $H_2O = H_2CO_3$, carbonic acid; also, there can be increases in interstitial lactic acid)

Arterioles are embedded within the interstitium of organs and their smooth muscle is affected by interstitial chemical constituents. The changes in interstitial constituents, described above, cause arteriolar smooth muscle relaxation and vasodilation.

An increase in organ work results in increased cell metabolism. Cell oxygen consumption increases and there is a fall in intracellular and interstitial PO_2. More ATP is split in a harder working cell and AMP, an ATP breakdown product, diffuses out of the cell. Enzymes in the interstitial fluid act on AMP to produce adenosine. Lactic acid is released from harder working cells as is CO_2 and interstitial pH decreases. Remember, the interstitium contains water and $CO_2 + H_2O \leftrightarrow H_2CO_3$, carbonic acid. Repeated action potentials result in more K^+ in the interstitial fluid from K^+ efflux with repeated repolarization. Decreased interstitial O_2 and pH and increased adenosine and K^+ have a combined effect of inducing relaxation of arteriolar smooth muscle and increasing organ blood flow. The harder the organ works, the more relaxed the arterioles become and the more blood flow increases.

An increase in organ blood flow brings more O_2 to the harder working tissue. Also, the increased blood flow carries away some of the interstitial PCO_2, lactic acid, and adenosine, and thereby, increases interstitial pH. Some of the K^+, adenosine, and any other vasodilatory factors that may be present are carried away in the increased blood flow. The result is that blood flow increases to a steady state level that is appropriate for the level of organ work. When organ work decreases, the above changes are reversed and organ blood flow decreases to settle at a new, lower steady state level.

Note, this is local feedback control and does not involve hormones or nerves. Local metabolic control is important, for example, in the brain, heart, and skeletal muscle. It is also present in the gut.

There is a good deal of uncertainty about the relative importance of each of the factors noted above in metabolic control. For instance, adenosine appears to play an important role when ischemia occurs. Ischemia, a reduction in blood flow below normal levels, does result in increased adenosine in ischemic tissue interstitium and adenosine does then induce vasodilation that mitigates some of the ischemia problem. However, evidence for adenosine playing a role in normal metabolic control is not consistent. Clearly, blood flow increases when work increases in an organ with local metabolic control, but the precise mechanisms remain to be worked out.

AUTOREGULATION

According to Poiseuille's law, the amount of blood flow is partly dependent on the difference of downstream mean pressure ($\bar{P}_2$) from upstream mean pressure ($\bar{P}_1$):

$$Q = \frac{\pi(\bar{P}_1 - \bar{P}_2)r^4}{8L\eta}$$

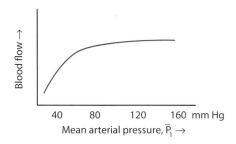

Figure 12.8 Autoregulation of organ blood flow. Steady state blood flow is plotted.

If downstream venous pressure ($\overline{P}_1$) does not change, then flow in an organ, Q, will increase with an increase in upstream, arterial mean pressure ($\overline{P}_2$). This will be true assuming nothing else changes in Poiseuille's law. However, when "autoregulation" is present, something else does change.

First, consider blood flow to an organ, such as the brain, whose circulation does manifest autoregulation. In this example, nothing has been done to alter vascular smooth muscle function in the organ (Figure 12.8). Blood flow increases with an increase in mean arterial pressure, $\overline{P}_1$, but only at very low pressures (Figure 12.8). Above approximately 60 mmHg mean arterial blood pressure there is little change in steady state blood flow (Figure 12.8).

An acute increase in mean arterial pressure does induce a transient increase in cerebral blood flow, not shown in Figure 12.8. But more blood entering the arterioles dilates them and stretches their walls. The arterioles in organs with autoregulation have smooth myocytes that are activated by stretch. Stretch of the arteriolar wall smooth muscle cells opens L-type Ca^{2+} channels and the smooth muscle contractions, vessel radius decreases and flow then decreases back close to where it was before. Steady state blood flow is little changed (Figure 12.8). In the context of Poiseuille's law, $\overline{P}_1$ increases, resulting in an increase in Q and arteriolar r^4, followed by arteriolar smooth muscle contraction, a decrease in r^4, and a return of Q toward its original level (Figure 12.8).

The transient rise in flow is not illustrated in Figure 12.2—the graph shows only steady state blood flow. This is one mechanism that explains, in the face of changing mean arterial pressure, the constancy of blood flow called autoregulation that is present in some organs.

Also, the transient initial increase in cerebral blood flow caused by an increase in mean arterial pressure increases cerebral interstitial PO_2 and washes away interstitial PCO_2. The transient increase in blood flow carries away adenosine, H^+, and K^+ that may be present. This vasodilator washout reduces arteriolar dilation and, with arteriolar smooth muscle stretch activation, nudges cerebral blood flow back toward where it had been prior to the increase in mean arterial pressure.

The vasodilator washout and myogenic mechanisms are both important. Caution! The fact that there is a chemical mechanism at work in autoregulation does not mean autoregulation is the same as local metabolic control. Local metabolic control matches blood flow to organ metabolism. Autoregulation acts to maintain constancy of flow. Brain, heart, kidney, and skeletal muscle are examples of organs with autoregulation.

Next, consider blood flow to the brain in an experiment where the arteriolar smooth muscle has been paralyzed with a drug. Now blood flow changes directly with mean arterial pressure. Autoregulation has been eliminated. This type of experiment highlights the importance of the myogenic mechanism of autoregulation.

Autoregulation also works with a fall in arterial mean blood pressure. Cerebral blood flow decreases transiently when arterial pressure decreases. The transiently reduced cerebral blood flow results in less stretch of the arteriolar walls. With less stretch vascular smooth myocytes relax and r^4 increases. Flow then increases to close to what it was before arterial pressure decreased. Likewise, with less flow there is less vasodilator washout of adenosine, CO_2, K^+, and lactic acid.

Autoregulation is not a reflex. There are no nerves or hormones involved. It is local control of organ blood flow inherent in blood vessel smooth muscle stretch activation and related to vasodilator washout from the interstitium.

ARTERIAL BLOOD PRESSURE AND SALT AND WATER METABOLISM

Arterial blood pressure is partially dependent on the amount of blood in the aorta. That is why stroke volume, vessel elasticity, and peripheral resistance are among the important determinants of blood pressure. Also of importance is the total volume and distribution of blood in the circulation. For instance, if total blood volume increases, the following sequence can occur:

- ↑ Total blood volume
- ↑ Aorta radius and circumference
- ↑ Stretch of the aorta
- ↑ Aorta wall tension
- ↑ Aortic blood pressure

The most common cardiovascular disease in the United States and many other countries is high blood pressure or hypertension. The etiology in most patients is unknown and the pathophysiology may not be the same in all patients. Some of the patients do have abnormalities in salt and water metabolism whereby total body sodium and water are greater than normal. Na^+ and the water accompanying it are distributed within the extracellular space, throughout the intravascular and interstitial compartments. The severity of high blood pressure in these patients is linked to their sodium intake. In these patients and in most other patients with high blood pressure, blood pressure is lowered to some degree by drugs that induce the kidneys to excrete sodium and water.

In summary, salt and water metabolism is important in the long-term control of systemic blood pressure levels. Although the mechanisms are complex, the important factors are clear and include the volume of the aorta (radius, circumference, and wall stretch) and aortic wall elasticity.

VEINS IN CIRCULATORY CONTROL

Veins are very distensible (compliant); consequently about 2/3 of circulating blood volume is in the venous part of the circulation. Blood flowing into veins easily distends the veins and increases their volume. The sympathetic nervous system is the primary controller of venous tone in some parts of the circulation, for instance, the kidney and splanchnic regions.

Increased lower body venous tone due to sympathetic stimulation of vascular alpha receptors enhances the return of blood to the right atrium during the baroreflex response to standing and helps to partially overcome the effects of gravity.

BLOOD PRESSURE CONTROL, THE AUTONOMIC NERVOUS SYSTEM, AND HEART FAILURE

Abnormalities in blood pressure control have been demonstrated in patients with heart failure. When compared with normal, the increase in heart rate with upright tilt is blunted. In some heart failure patients there is a significant drop in blood pressure as compared with normal during upright tilt. The mechanisms are not totally clear. One factor may be a down-regulation of myocardial beta receptors and reduced norepinephrine synthesis in cardiac sympathetic nerve endings in heart failure.

Heart failure, even in the early stages, is accompanied by increases above normal in circulating norepinephrine and sometimes epinephrine as well. Increased sympathetic activity accounts for higher heart rates in heart failure patients. The renin-angiotensin-aldosterone system is activated by increased sympathetic activity. More sympathetic activity and more angiotensin II lead to widespread vasoconstriction, a hallmark of heart failure.

There is evidence that catecholamines and angiotensin II influences on myocardial myocytes enhance development of myocardial hypertrophy and proliferation of embryonic proteins. These cellular and molecular changes are called adverse remodeling. There is then a vicious cycle of reduced ventricular function in heart failure leading to more proliferation of abnormal myocyte proteins leading to more compromise of function. Beta blocking agents and angiotensin converting enzyme inhibitors or angiotensin II receptor blocking drugs are used in heart failure treatment, in large part to reduce deleterious myocardial remodeling.

Pathophysiological changes in neural and hormonal control systems in heart failure are illustrated in the self-study module Myocardial Infarction and Chronic Heart Failure.

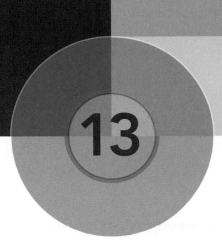

Regional blood flow

INTRODUCTION

The control of blood flow to regions varies. There is perhaps no better illustration of this than dynamic exercise on a stationary bicycle or treadmill. Splanchnic and renal blood flow decrease with such exercise simultaneous with a substantial increase in coronary and skeletal muscle blood flow, and cerebral blood flow hardly changes at all. Regional blood flow also can alter with disease. It is apparent that it is essential to understand regional controls of blood flow.

CEREBRAL BLOOD FLOW

There are four arteries that deliver almost all the blood to the brain: bilateral internal carotid and vertebral arteries. The two vertebral arteries join to form the basilar artery. There is a minor contribution from the anterior spinal artery. Venous outflow is via the internal jugular and vertebral veins.

REGULATION OF CEREBRAL BLOOD FLOW: POISEUILLE'S LAW

Factors that determine cerebral blood flow are noted in Figure 13.1. These factors are the variables in Poiseuille's law. L, length, of brain blood vessels does not change except with maturation. There is the additional factor of intracranial pressure that will be discussed.

ARTERIOLAR RADIUS

The sympathetic nervous system plays a small role in normal control of the cerebral vasculature. For instance, there are few α receptors on cerebral arteries or arterioles and sympathetic-induced vasoconstriction is minimal. Cerebral arteries are innervated by vasodilating perivascular C-fiber nerves and parasympathetic nerves that play a role in the pathophysiology of migraine headaches, but have a limited role in controlling cerebral blood flow.

Cerebral blood flow is influenced by the PCO_2 of arterial blood (Figure 13.2). CO_2 is lipid soluble and readily diffuses across brain capillaries. An increase in arterial PCO_2 decreases the gradient across the capillary wall for CO_2 diffusion out of the brain, brain interstitial fluid PCO_2 increases, and pH decreases (Figure 13.2). Arterioles in the brain, as in all organs, are embedded within the brain interstitial tissue and the arteriolar smooth muscle is sensitive to interstitial fluid pH (Figure 13.2). PCO_2 combines with interstitial water to form H_2CO_3 (Figure 13.2). The

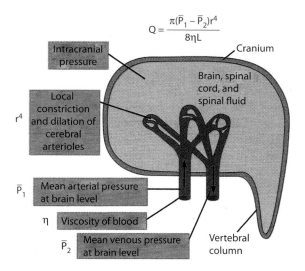

$$Q = \frac{\pi(\bar{P}_1 - \bar{P}_2)r^4}{8\eta L}$$

Figure 13.1 Factors important in brain blood flow. (Adapted from Barrett KE et al. *Ganong's Review of Medical Physiology*, 23rd ed. New York, NY: McGraw-Hill; 2010. With permission of McGraw-Hill.)

lower brain tissue pH results in relaxation of arteriolar smooth muscle, vasodilatation (Figure 13.1, increase in r^4), and more cerebral blood flow (Figure 13.2).

The converse of the above occurs if arterial PCO_2 decreases. For instance, if one were to breathe in and out deeply and rapidly enough to blow off more CO_2 than is produced in the body, arterial PCO_2 decreases. A decrease in arterial PCO_2 due to rapid breathing is defined as hyperventilation. The decrease in arterial PCO_2 increases the concentration gradient across the capillary wall from the brain interstitium to the blood and more PCO_2 leaves the brain (Figure 13.2). This results in interstitial brain alkalosis, cerebral arteriolar constriction, and a decrease in cerebral blood flow (Figure 13.2). Dizziness and syncope due to decreased cerebral blood flow can occur.

Note: The level of blood pH has negligible effects on brain blood flow because H^+ and OH^- ions in the blood do not readily cross the capillary walls in the brain. The blood–brain barrier is discussed below.

MEAN ARTERIAL PRESSURE

Cerebral hypoxia due to inadequate cerebral blood flow develops below a mean arterial blood pressure of 60 mm Hg. There is autoregulation of cerebral blood flow that operates above this arterial blood pressure level, as discussed above.

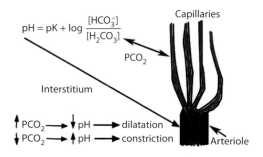

Figure 13.2 Influence of arterial PCO_2 and brain interstitial pH on brain blood flow.

MEAN VENOUS PRESSURE

BLOOD VISCOSITY

Mean venous pressure and blood viscosity have been discussed earlier in Chapter 8, How the Circulation Works and in Chapter 11, Peripheral Circulation, Poiseuille's law.

REGULATION OF CEREBRAL BLOOD FLOW: INTRACRANIAL PRESSURE

The adult central nervous system lies within a rigid container, the skull and vertebral column (Figure 13.1). The brain, spinal cord, cerebrospinal fluid, and cerebral vessels normally fill this rigid container. Since the total capacity is fixed, any increase in the volume of any component within the central nervous system must result in an increase in intracranial pressure and compression of other components. An increase in intracranial pressure constitutes an increase in external pressure on the central nervous system blood vessels. An increase in intracranial pressure squeezes the intracranial blood vessels and reduces their radius.

One complication of a brain tumor is increased intracranial pressure. As the tumor grows, intracranial pressure increases. Arterial inflow to the brain is reduced because of the increased intracranial pressure and decreased blood vessel radius (r^4) (Figure 13.1). The decrease in r^4 constitutes an increase in cerebral vascular resistance. Therefore, inadequate cerebral blood flow (cerebral ischemia) can be an added problem in such a patient.

CHANGES IN CEREBRAL BLOOD FLOW

Blood PCO_2 is tightly regulated by the respiratory system and normally remains constant even during mild to moderate exercise. The constant blood PCO_2 and autoregulation result in mostly constant brain blood flow. Overall brain metabolism is for the most part constant and changes little with the transition, for instance, from intense mental activity to relaxation.

But there is a change in local brain blood flow with local activity. Increases in local blood flow come about because of more brain nerve cell activity and local metabolic control. Also, as elsewhere in the circulation, endothelial vasoactive factors partly control the vasculature.

Brain astrocytes surround and communicate with neurons, and have a role in neuronal metabolism. The end-feet of astrocytes contact neuronal cell bodies and arterioles and release neurotransmitter substances that are vasoactive, such as NO. This is another mechanism for linking local increases in neuronal activity with local vasodilation.

SUMMARY OF CEREBRAL BLOOD FLOW REGULATION

Arterial blood levels	Brain circulation
$\uparrow PCO_2$	Vasodilatation
$\downarrow PCO_2$	Vasoconstriction
$\uparrow$ or $\downarrow$ pH (pH here is arterial blood pH, not brain interstitial pH)	Minor effects (H^+ and OH^- do not easily cross the blood–brain barrier, discussed below)

Local metabolic control—brain cell release of lactic acid, K^+, CO_2, and adenosine. Also, astrocytes and local vasoactive substances play a role.

The autonomic nervous system innervates larger cerebral arteries, but has a minor influence on the control of cerebral blood flow.

Autoregulation is important.

BLOOD–BRAIN BARRIER

Endothelial cell junctions in most of the adult brain capillaries are tight and have few if any pores. Diffusion between blood and the brain interstitium is very limited in most of the brain tissue. Astrocytes, surround the cerebral blood vessels and play a role in limiting diffusion between the brain interstitium and blood.

As is true in capillaries elsewhere, lipid soluble materials (O_2, CO_2, ethanol, and anesthetics) dissolve through the endothelial wall. Diffusion rates and transport mechanisms in brain capillaries are different from capillaries in other parts of the circulation. Catecholamines do not readily pass the barrier and brain blood vessel endothelium contains monoamine oxidase that breaks down catecholamines. As noted below, there is a carrier system for glucose in the capillary membrane. Other materials (heavy metals, antibiotics) pass the barrier with difficulty compared with capillary beds in other parts of the body. Consideration of the blood–brain barrier becomes important, for example, when selecting drugs to treat a brain infection or if a toxin is present in the bloodstream.

Some fetal red blood cells normally cross the placenta into the maternal blood stream. If an Rh− mother has an Rh+ baby, the maternal blood develops antibodies that diffuse across the placenta and destroy the baby's red blood cells. Hemoglobin released from the damaged fetal red blood cells is metabolized by the fetal liver and results in a rise in blood levels of bile pigments. The newborn immature blood–brain barrier does allow bile pigments to pass across into the brain. The bile pigments cross the immature blood–brain barrier and can cause brain damage. Brain damage of this type is not a problem in adult liver disease or hemolytic anemia because there is full development of the adult blood–brain barrier to bile pigments.

BRAIN METABOLISM

Glucose is the major energy source for the brain and there is a carrier-mediated transfer of glucose across the blood–brain barrier. A major complication of hypoglycemia, such as with excessive insulin in a diabetic, is brain cell dysfunction and convulsions.

LYMPHATIC DRAINAGE

The role of lymphatic drainage of brain tissue is being investigated. Cerebral lymphatic drainage is limited. Cerebral spinal fluid does equilibrate with blood via capillaries in some locations in the arachnoid sinuses and there may be lymphatic vessels originating in arachnoid tissue.

CORONARY BLOOD FLOW

ANATOMY

The two main coronary arteries arise from the sinus of Valsalva of the anterior right and left aortic valve cusps (Figure 13.3). Coronary artery orifices are patent throughout the cardiac cycle

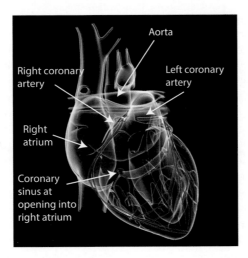

Figure 13.3 Coronary artery anatomy.

because a small amount of normal turbulence at the cusps during ejection keeps the aortic valve leaflets from flattening against the sinus walls.

The main arteries and their major branches are on the surface of the ventricles. Branches emerge at right angles to these main vessels and penetrate the ventricular wall. The right-angle branches arborize into small arteries, arterioles, and so on, all within the ventricular muscular wall.

CORONARY BLOOD FLOW AND FLOW DEPENDENT OXYGEN SUPPLY

At rest, aortic blood O_2 content is about 20 mL O_2/100 mL blood. Pulmonary artery blood O_2 content is typically about 15 mL/100 mL blood. Therefore, the tissues of the entire body extract from the systemic circulation about 5 mL O_2/100 mL blood. In contrast, the O_2 content of coronary sinus venous blood in a normal heart is 5 mL O_2/100 mL blood. Coronary sinus blood flow is the major venous effluent from the left ventricle. The left ventricular myocardium then extracts about 15 mL O_2/100 mL blood or roughly 3 times the O_2 extraction per unit of blood as compared with the rest of the body. Even in a normal heart in a resting individual, most of the oxygen is being extracted from blood passing through the coronary circulation. This fact leads to an extremely important clinical concept:

> An increase in coronary blood flow is the major way the oxygen supply to heart muscle can be increased. The capacity for increasing O_2 extraction from coronary blood flow is very limited.

This is what is meant by a flow-dependent oxygen supply. For instance, consider a patient who has a partially obstructed coronary artery and you will appreciate the problem that can arise when more myocardial O_2 is needed, such as during exercise. The partial obstruction can limit the increase in coronary blood flow during exercise. Since O_2 extraction is close to maximum before exercise begins, extraction of more oxygen from the coronary blood flow during exercise is limited. The result may be failure to supply enough of an increase in coronary blood flow to supply the increased O_2 demand of the exercising heart.

CONTROL OF CORONARY BLOOD FLOW

The amount of coronary blood flow is determined primarily by local metabolic control. A change in cardiac work, due to an increase in heart rate, pressure development, or both is the major driver of metabolic change and coronary blood flow.

Sympathetic and to some extent parasympathetic nerves innervate coronary arterioles. Sympathetic stimulation of beta receptors on arterioles contributes about 25% of the total arteriolar vasodilation during exercise or stress, the rest being due to local metabolic control. There also is sympathetic stimulation of alpha receptors on larger coronary arteries. The resulting activation of medium and large size coronary artery smooth muscle reduces their expansion with increased flow and enhances forward blood movement. Nervous influences also probably play a role in maintaining basal arteriolar smooth muscle tone.

Secondary to, for instance, excitement or exercise, the rate of firing of action potentials increases along sympathetic nerves to the sinus node and ventricular muscle. Heart rate increases as does the rate and extent of force development and shortening of heart muscle fibers. Stroke volume increases. Systolic blood pressure increases. Myocardial work increases because heart rate increases and systolic ventricular pressure is higher. Myocardial metabolism increases and coronary blood flow increases primarily because of local metabolic control.

It is increased cardiac work and an associated increase in myocardial oxygen consumption brought on by sympathetic stimulation that brings about approximately 75% of the coronary arteriolar dilatation and increased coronary blood flow. Direct nervous control of the coronary vasculature accounts for the remaining 25%.

CORONARY BLOOD FLOW, WORK RELATIONSHIP

If ventricular pressure or wall tension increases, myocardial metabolism increases and blood flow increases due primarily to local metabolic control. Anything that increases the amount of myocardial pressure work will increase myocardial metabolism, significantly dilate coronary arterioles, and increase the amount of coronary blood flow. Coronary blood flow is then linked to the myocardial need for O_2 via local metabolic control.

MAJOR DETERMINANTS OF MYOCARDIAL OXYGEN CONSUMPTION

The major determinants of coronary blood flow are those factors that strongly influence systolic wall tension (tension is force per unit length) per unit time:

- *Intraventricular pressure development*: Ventricular pressure development is a major determinant of myocardial oxygen consumption.
- *Ventricular size and configuration (law of Laplace)*: Ventricular wall tension during systole is a major determinant of myocardial O_2 consumption. Systolic wall tension is the force in the ventricular wall produced by the myocytes. Wall tension is directly related to pressure via the law of Laplace, $P = (T/r)$. This simplified version of the formula can be rearranged to $T = Pr$. In a dilated ventricle (large r) the amount of ventricular wall tension (T) to produce a given intraventricular pressure is greater than in a ventricle that is not dilated. This becomes important in a patient with, for instance, heart failure or dilated cardiomyopathy. The version of Laplace's law applied to a ventricle is

$$T = \frac{Pr}{2h}$$

The h is wall thickness. In, for instance, hypertrophy resulting from aortic valvular stenosis, left ventricular pressure, P, increases, but so does wall thickness, h. Since there is more muscle tissue, pressure development is shared by more muscle and wall tension is less than it would otherwise be. The increase in h helps to minimize the increase in T. As the aortic valve narrows and left ventricular pressure, P, continues to climb, T does increase despite h increasing and myocardial O_2 demands increase. One complication of aortic valvular stenosis is exercise-induced ischemia due to demand for O_2 exceeding supply.

- *Heart rate*: No surprise here—every heartbeat consumes O_2 and O_2 consumption increases as heart rate increases.
- *Contractility*: An increase in contractility is accompanied by more vigorous ventricular contraction with a likely increase in pulmonary artery and aortic pressure. The ventricles work harder and require more O_2.

MINOR DETERMINANTS OF MYOCARDIAL OXYGEN CONSUMPTION

There are several minor determinants of myocardial oxygen consumption that play less of a role in determining coronary blood flow:

- *Stroke volume*: Stroke volume production occurs due to ventricular wall myocyte shortening, but consumes relatively little O_2 in addition to that producing force development.
- *Activation energy*: ATP used in depolarization and excitation-contraction coupling is in this category and is a relatively small quantity.

AUTOREGULATION

There is autoregulation in the coronary vasculature. Autoregulation becomes particularly important when blood pressure falls in the coronary vasculature distal to a coronary artery obstruction. The fall in blood pressure reduces wall stretch, the coronary arteriolar smooth muscle relaxes, and the radius increases. Autoregulation then partially offsets the reduction of flow distal to the obstruction.

CORONARY BLOOD FLOW AND THE CARDIAC CYCLE

SYSTOLE

Coronary arterial inflow varies during the cardiac cycle, particularly in the left ventricle (Figure 13.4). Intramyocardial coronary arterial vessels are squeezed by contracting myocardium during systole. Reduction of vessel radius and the attendant increase in coronary vascular resistance results in reduced coronary arterial inflow during systole (shaded portion of graph in Figure 13.4). Aortic pressure is high enough during left ventricular ejection to drive some blood through the elevated coronary vascular resistance. The variations in blood flow are less pronounced in the lower pressure, thinner-walled right ventricle (Figure 13.4).

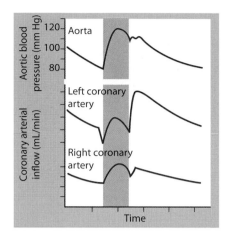

Figure 13.4 Variations in coronary arterial inflow during the cardiac cycle.

DIASTOLE

Most coronary artery inflow occurs during diastole (Figure 13.4) when the myocardium is relaxed. This is particularly true in the left ventricle because of the greater variation in pressure levels and wall tension than in the right ventricle. When heart rate increases in exercise, the duration of diastole decreases much more than the duration of systole. The time available for coronary arterial inflow decreases. This is not a problem for a normal person because the extent of coronary arteriolar vasodilation caused by the increased cardiac work and local metabolic control results in adequate coronary blood flow.

Tachycardia occurring in a patient with coronary artery narrowing or with an abnormally increased demand for coronary blood flow, like a patient with aortic stenosis, can result in inadequate coronary blood flow relative to the metabolic demands of the heart.

VENOUS OUTFLOW

Venous outflow increases during systole. Ventricular muscle contraction squeezes veins and propels venous blood through the coronary sinus and other veins. There is much less squeeze during diastole and veins fill before the next systole. Venous outflow is not included in Figure 13.4.

ENDOTHELIAL VASOACTIVE FACTORS

Control of coronary blood flow related to endothelial vasoactive factors is important. Changes in coronary blood vessel endothelial cell function are proving to be important in understanding coronary heart disease.

CLINICAL CASE

An 85-year-old man has been having gradually increasing difficulty with shortness of breath with exertion over the past 6 months. Also, he has experienced pressure-like anterior chest pain in the last week with climbing a flight of stairs. On several occasions in the past 5 years he has been told of having a heart murmur and there is a systolic ejection murmur present (discussed earlier in Chapter 9, Cardiac Cycle, Heart Sounds and Murmurs [Figure 9.8]). What is the heart murmur due to? What is the etiology of the chest pain?

> **This patient has aortic valvular stenosis, which is presented in the self-study module Cardiac Cycle: Heart Sounds and Murmurs.** His left ventricle is likely hypertrophied and more muscle requires more O_2. Also, left ventricular blood pressure and wall tension, major determinants of myocardial O_2 demand, are higher than normal and increase further with exercise. The chest pain is likely related to exertional myocardial ischemia. Myocardial work during his exertion increases myocardial O_2 consumption enough to exceed O_2 delivery by the coronary blood flow. Of course, his doctors will have to exclude the presence of any coronary artery partial obstructions.

e

SKELETAL MUSCLE BLOOD FLOW

ANATOMICAL AND MECHANICAL CONSIDERATIONS

Skeletal muscle arterial blood inflow decreases during contraction as arterial branches between muscle bundles are squeezed. In exercise, such as jogging, leg skeletal muscles alternately contract and relax with the rhythmic movement of the legs. Arterial inflow decreases during contraction and increases with relaxation. During such exercise, overall skeletal muscle blood flow increases due to the extent of arteriolar vasodilatation brought about by local metabolic control.

Skeletal muscle contraction squeezes veins within the muscle bundles. Valves in the veins in the lower extremities open toward the right atrium and prevent reflux back toward the muscle when the muscle relaxes. The rhythmic contraction and relaxation of leg skeletal muscles acts as a pump, the skeletal muscle pump discussed earlier (Chapter 10, Ventricular Function). The venous vascular bed fills from the arterial side during relaxation and during muscle contraction blood in the veins is pushed toward the heart. The direction is one-way due to the venous valves. This skeletal muscle pump phenomenon becomes important for venous return to the right atrium during upright dynamic exercise such as running or bicycling.

SKELETAL MUSCLE BLOOD FLOW CONTROL

LOCAL METABOLIC CONTROL

Arterioles in working, contracting skeletal muscles are predominately under local metabolic control rather than autonomic nervous system control.

SYMPATHETIC EFFECTS

Arterioles in resting skeletal muscle are under the direct control of the sympathetic nervous system and circulating catecholamines. Constriction of resting skeletal muscle arterioles is part of the baroreceptor mechanism that is important in maintaining blood pressure when standing upright at rest. This vasoconstriction is due to release of norepinephrine at sympathetic nerves ending on arteriolar myocyte α receptors. Resting skeletal muscle blood flow is reduced during intense sympathetic stimulation such as in a patient with advanced heart failure or hypovolemic shock due to blood loss.

Beta adrenergic receptors (β_2) are present in skeletal muscle arterioles. Arterioles dilate in response to low levels of circulating epinephrine as a balance to the α receptor activity. This type of vasodilation may be important in low level exercise. During higher levels of exercise local metabolic control predominates.

OXYGEN DELIVERY

Interstitial pH drops and temperature rises due to the metabolic activity of mechanically active muscle. Increased acidic metabolites such as lactate and CO_2 contribute to a decrease in interstitial fluid pH. Lactic acid enters the blood and results in a drop in arterial pH during moderate to heavy exercise.

The heat of muscle work warms blood as it circulates through a muscle. Also, core body temperature rises after about 5 minutes of a sustained bout of dynamic exercise. Gradually, all blood in the body is warmed and the temperature of arterial blood entering working muscles increases.

Drop in blood pH and rise in blood temperature result in an increase in blood PO_2 at any given level of O_2 saturation. At any given level of saturation, warmed acidic hemoglobin more readily releases O_2. This assists in O_2 delivery to working muscles.

AUTOREGULATION

Autoregulation is present in resting skeletal muscle. Autoregulation is overridden by metabolic factors during muscle mechanical activity.

PULMONARY BLOOD FLOW

Pulmonary vascular resistance normally is less than a tenth of systemic vascular resistance. Pulmonary arterioles are shorter and have less smooth muscle than in the systemic circulation. Pulmonary vascular resistance is less localized than in the systemic circulation. Resistance is distributed among the small arteries, arterioles, and the microvasculature, including the venules. Also, the pulmonary vasculature is exposed to a low level of external pressure because of the spongy lung tissue and negative (below atmospheric) intrathoracic pressure.

CHARACTERISTICS OF PULMONARY BLOOD FLOW

There is very little extravascular support. Lung tissue is spongy. Small pulmonary arteries, arterioles, capillaries, and venules form a meshwork within the alveolar walls. They are intrapulmonic. The larger Pulmonary arteries and veins are largely free of surrounding pulmonary tissue. They are extrapulmonic. As noted above, external pressure on all these vessels is low because intrathoracic pressure is below atmospheric.

In a resting person, during inspiration, external pressure on the extrapulmonic arteries and veins decreases further. However, intrapulmonic vessels are "squeezed" by expanding alveoli, the radius of these vessels decreases and pulmonary vascular resistance rises, although it is still far less than systemic vascular resistance.

With very deep inspiration in a resting person, intrapulmonary blood vessels are stretched. L increases and r decreases, which acts to impede blood flow. Remember:

$$\text{F or Q} = \frac{\pi(\bar{P}_1 - \bar{P}_2)r^4}{8\eta L}$$

Local control of pulmonary blood flow is predominantly related to alveolar air PO_2. In regions where alveolar air PO_2 is low the local arterioles constrict. The site of this vasoconstriction is in precapillary sphincters and arterioles. If in an experiment alveolar air PO_2 is reduced and pulmonary artery blood PO_2 is increased, pulmonary vasoconstriction does occur. Therefore, the primary factor controlling pulmonary arteriolar caliber appears to be the alveolar air PO_2 rather than pulmonary artery blood PO_2.

There is controversy regarding the factors mediating vasoconstriction resulting from a drop in alveolar air PO_2. Histamine, angiotensin, and catecholamines all have been implicated, but a specific mediator is not known. A drop in alveolar air PO_2 does result in decreased pH of the local lung tissue. Lung tissue acidosis causes vasoconstriction, not dilatation, as is the case in other parts of the circulation.

Finally, hypoxia inhibits a K^+ current in pulmonary vascular smooth muscle. The resulting depolarization of the smooth muscle cells opens Ca^{2+} channels and the influx of Ca^{2+} induces contraction and vasoconstriction. Experimental evidence is not completely satisfactory for any one explanation of the mechanism whereby alveolar air hypoxia induces pulmonary vasoconstriction.

It may seem disadvantageous for flow to decrease with alveolar hypoxia. However, consider a situation in which a bronchial branch is obstructed. That segment of the lung is not aerated and alveolar PO_2 falls. Vasoconstriction in that segment diverts blood away from the poorly ventilated alveoli to better aerated alveoli with normal PO_2 levels and thereby preserves the relationship of ventilation with perfusion.

There are sympathetic and parasympathetic nerve fibers to the lung, and there are α and β receptors on small artery and arteriolar smooth muscle cells. However, the influence of the autonomic nervous system on the pulmonary vasculature is minimal. Although sympathetic nerve activity increases in, for instance, exercise, the overwhelming response in the pulmonary circulation is passive dilatation and reduced vascular resistance in exercise. There are major autonomic influences on bronchial smooth muscle, which will not be discussed here.

Endothelial vasoactive factors play a critical role here as in the coronary and other circulations. Angiotensin II can cause some vasoconstriction in small arteries and arterioles in the lung.

CHANGES WITH POSTURE AND DYNAMIC EXERCISE

In upright posture, blood pressure in the apical vasculature is lower than in the base due to gravitational, hydrostatic effects. Transmural pressure (pressure inside the blood vessel minus pressure outside) is low in the apical vasculature, the blood vessel radius is then small and vascular resistance is high. Thus, in the upright posture there is a vertical gradation of blood flow in the lung, lowest in the apex and highest in the base.

There is a modest increase in pulmonary artery mean pressure during upright dynamic exercise, even with large increases in cardiac output (CO). Therefore, pulmonary vascular resistance must have decreased concomitant with the increase in pulmonary blood flow. Remember:

$$CO = \frac{\overline{P}_1 - \overline{P}_2}{R}$$

$\overline{P}_1$ is mean pulmonary artery and $\overline{P}_2$ is mean left atrial blood pressure. If $\overline{P}_1$ increases less than expected with the increase in CO, then R, pulmonary vascular resistance, must have decreased.

There are several mechanisms for the decrease in pulmonary vascular resistance during dynamic exercise.

As pulmonary blood flow increases, pressure increases within the pulmonary blood vessels. Any increase in intravascular pulmonary arterial pressure results in an increase in blood vessel radius. Pulmonary blood vessel smooth muscle is not stretch activated and there is no autoregulation. Therefore, the increase in radius reduces resistance and blunts the tendency for pulmonary artery pressure to increase.

As described above, in an upright resting person perfusion of blood vessels in the lung apices is reduced because of the effects of gravity. During upright exercise the modest increase in pressure in the pulmonary vasculature is enough to overcome some of the effects of gravity and increase apical lung blood flow. Blood vessels in the lung apices not fully opened at rest are further opened by the increased pulmonary arterial blood pressure. There is then recruitment of parallel blood vessels during upright exercise and that contributes to reduced pulmonary vascular resistance.

RENAL BLOOD FLOW

There are two sets of arterioles in series. The first set of arterioles, the pre-glomerular or afferent arterioles, control blood flow into the capillary network of the glomeruli. The second set, the efferent arterioles, control blood flow into the rest of the kidney capillaries. All the kidney arteriolar myocytes are richly innervated by sympathetic fibers. Afferent arteriole myocytes are innervated by sympathetic nerves ending on α-receptors. Sympathetic stimulation results in vasoconstriction and can lead to a reduction in overall renal blood flow. Constriction of post-glomerular arterioles during sympathetic stimulation will tend to raise glomerular hydrostatic pressure and enhance glomerular filtration.

Kidney arterioles manifest autoregulation. There is relatively constant renal blood flow (RBF) with arterial mean blood pressure levels of 70 to 170 mm Hg and glomerular filtration rate stays constant over this range. This tendency for stability of renal blood flow contributes to optimizing renal function. In addition to the mechanisms of autoregulation described earlier, in the kidney there is tubuloglomerular feedback. An increase in kidney blood flow and glomerular capillary blood pressure transiently result in more glomerular filtration. More water and Na^+ are filtered, travel through the renal tubules, and the increased tubular Na^+ is sensed by the macula densa. This leads to vasoconstriction of the afferent arteriole and a return of blood flow and filtration close to their original levels. The combination of tubuloglomerular feedback and stretch activation of vascular smooth muscle maintains stability of renal blood flow and glomerular filtration.

The renin-angiotensin system and the participation of the kidney in control of the circulation is discussed in Chapter 12, Circulatory Controls.

GASTROINTESTINAL BLOOD FLOW

The spleen-to-liver and gut-to-liver vasculature are examples of sets of arterioles and capillaries in series, as in the kidney. Autoregulation is not a prominent feature, but control by the sympathetic nervous system is. Arteriolar myocytes have α-receptors and vasoconstriction is a prominent feature of sympathetic activity, such as during dynamic exercise. Vasodilatation occurs in response to local metabolic activity, as with digestion. Vasodilatation in response to vagal stimulation is probably indirectly due to increased gut activity.

CUTANEOUS BLOOD FLOW

Cutaneous blood flow plays an essential role in the regulation of body temperature as well as in skin nutrition. Cutaneous blood flow most involved in body temperature control is in the skin in exposed parts of the body.

EXPOSURE TO A COLD ENVIRONMENT

Cold ambient temperatures result in cutaneous vasoconstriction due to a combination of three mechanisms.

- There is a direct effect of skin cooling on vascular smooth muscle. A moderate decrease in skin vascular smooth muscle temperature results in vasoconstriction.
- A second mechanism involves a nerve reflex. There is evidence for a nervous reflex from the skin to the hypothalamus via not well-defined afferent pathways. Efferent pathways from the hypothalamus result in sympathetic mediated vasoconstriction of arteriovenous anastomoses or metarterioles (Figure 13.5).
- Finally, a third mechanism is related to cooled venous blood returning from cooled skin. The cooled venous blood decreases the temperature of blood in the circulation. The hypothalamus has extremely sensitive temperature receptors and an extensive vasculature. A fraction of a degree change in blood temperature can be sensed by the hypothalamic temperature sensitive cells. The efferent pathway from the hypothalamus is over sympathetic nerves to α-receptors, particularly those innervating metarterioles (Figure 13.5, metarterioles, also called arteriovenous anastomoses). Vasoconstriction in the skin diverts blood away from the body surface, reduces heart loss, and acts to maintain a stable core body temperature in a cold ambient environment.

EXPOSURE TO A WARM ENVIRONMENT

Warm ambient temperatures result in cutaneous vasodilatation due to three mechanisms.

- There is a direct effect of skin warming on vascular smooth muscle. Warmed skin arteriolar smooth muscle is less responsive to norepinephrine-induced contraction. Also, there is more NO activity in warmed skin arterioles.
- A second mechanism involves decreased sympathetic vasoconstrictor activity. Warmer blood returning from the periphery raises circulating blood temperature. The hypothalamus is perfused with warmer blood and this induces a reduction in hypothalamic output over sympathetic nerves to arteriovenous anastomoses (Figure 13.5). The decreased

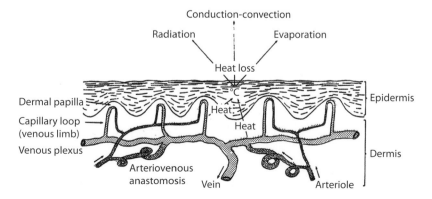

Figure 13.5 Cutaneous blood flow and temperature control. The vessels labeled "arteriovenous anastomosis" are metarterioles or thoroughfare channels. They are muscular vessels going from arteriole to venule. (From Levick JR. *An Introduction to Cardiovascular Physiology*, 5th ed. London, England: Hodder Arnold; 2011. With permission of Taylor and Francis.)

sympathetic activity to α-receptors results in passive arteriovenous dilatation and more skin blood flow.

- In the third mechanism there is increased nervous input to the hypothalamus from temperature sensors in the skin. This results in increased sympathetic cholinergic stimulation of sweat glands. Sweat gland activity results in sweat secreted onto the skin surface and the production of substances that diffuse into the skin interstitium. These substances act on interstitial fluid proteins to produce vasodilators. Bradykinin may be one such vasodilator.

Increased skin blood flow enhances heat loss by bringing warm blood to the body surface. Heat is then lost through radiation and conduction/convection. Evaporation of sweat on the skin surface also increases heat loss.

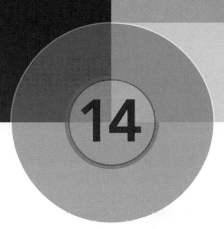

Microcirculation

The microcirculation consists of the arteriolar inflow to the capillary network, the capillary network and the venous outflow (Figure 14.1). Arterioles and venules have smooth muscle. Capillaries (Figure 14.1) consist of only endothelial cells.

ARTERIOLES

Blood flow from the arterial supply of an organ to its capillary bed is determined by the amount of constriction or dilatation of the small muscular arteries and arterioles. All tissues have arterioles (Figure 14.1). Some also have precapillary sphincters. Each precapillary sphincter is a circle of smooth muscle that surrounds the origin of a capillary from an arteriole (not pictured in Figure 14.1). These sphincters participate with arterioles in the control of blood entering the capillaries. When either an arteriole or a precapillary sphincter constricts, blood flow and pressure fall in the downstream capillaries. When they dilate, capillary blood flow and pressure increase.

CAPILLARIES

A capillary wall consists of a single layer of endothelial cells. Exchange is facilitated by the very high surface area to volume ratio in the capillary bed. Also, there is no muscle or connective tissue in capillary walls, the wall is thin and diffusion in and out is facilitated.

There are pores between adjacent endothelial cells in most of the microvasculature. Such pores are mostly small or absent in the adult cerebral circulation where a blood–brain barrier is present. Glomerular capillaries in the kidney act to filter the blood and their pores are prominent and highly specialized.

METARTERIOLES

Metarterioles are shunt vessels. Other names are "thoroughfare channel" and "arteriovenous anastomosis." They are present in certain specialized areas. As discussed above (Chapter 13, Regional Blood Flow), parts of the skin microcirculation are particularly rich in metarterioles. The increase in heat loss through the skin in response to an increase in ambient temperature is

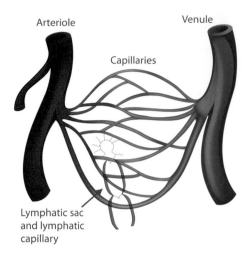

Figure 14.1 The microcirculation and lymphatics. (The superimposed illustration of a lymphatic vessel is from Levick JR. *An Introduction to Cardiovascular Physiology*, 5th ed. London, England: Hodder Arnold; 2011. With permission of Taylor & Francis Group.)

due largely to a reflex increase in cutaneous metarteriole blood flow (Figure 13.5 in Chapter 13, Regional Blood Flow, cutaneous blood flow). The increased cutaneous metarteriolar flow brings more blood to the body surface to facilitate heat loss. This flow is non-nutritional. It bypasses the capillary bed and shunts blood from the arterial to the venous side of the circulation. There is reflex metarteriolar constriction on exposure to cold ambient temperatures.

POSTCAPILLARY RESISTANCE

When venules (Figure 14.1) constrict, resistance to flow out of a capillary bed increases and capillary hydrostatic pressure and capillary filtration increase. Blood pressure in the kidney glomerular capillaries is partly dependent on the series resistance offered by the efferent arterioles.

The venous portion of the circulation accommodates a large blood volume—normally 60% to 70% of total blood volume resides there. Veins are thin-walled and relatively compliant and, as discussed earlier, readily expand as blood flows into them. The venous portion of the circulation characteristically has a large volume and low blood pressure.

NATURE OF BLOOD FLOW IN THE MICROCIRCULATION

NOT LAMINAR OR TURBULENT

Capillary blood flow is not laminar. Red blood cells (RBCs) move in single file because of the dimension of RBCs relative to the average capillary diameter: 8 μm vessel diameter and 2×8 μm RBCs. The biconcave RBCs must fold and slide through the capillary lumen. This minimizes diffusion distance from RBC to the interstitium. The flow is intermittent and dependent on arteriolar or precapillary sphincter control. There is no possibility for flow to be streamlined or turbulent as RBCs move in a single file with intervening plasma columns.

INTERMITTENT

When capillary blood flow is observed directly, such as in the mesenteric vessels of a frog or rat, it is seen to be intermittent. Blood flow in any one capillary can proceed forward, stop or reverse direction, and move slow or fast. Arteriolar control fluctuates in response, for instance, to local changes in metabolism. For example, in ventricular myocardium, the extent of constriction or relaxation of an arteriole is related to the metabolism of the myocytes that surround it.

SLOW

As discussed earlier, capillaries are the most numerous of blood vessels in the body. The flow of blood in each capillary is the slowest in the circulation. This is because the total cardiac output is divided among many millions of capillaries. Slow flow is optimal for diffusion and exchange.

FORCES DETERMINING TRANSCAPILLARY EXCHANGE

There is a complete presentation of transcapillary fluid movement in the self-study module Transcapillary Fluid Exchange: Starling Principle of Fluid Movement across a Capillary Wall.

e

- *Capillary blood pressure*: The blood pressure within a capillary, P_c, also called the hydrostatic pressure, is an important determinant of fluid transudation (Figure 14.2). As noted above, capillary blood pressure is determined by the combined effects of arteriolar and precapillary sphincter smooth muscle activity, mean venous pressure, and venular smooth muscle activity. A high ratio of postcapillary to precapillary resistance favors an increase in capillary blood pressure and more capillary filtration.

  If arteriolar and precapillary sphincter smooth muscle is relaxed and precapillary resistance is low, flow into and pressure within the capillaries will be greater than when precapillary resistance is high. An increase in postcapillary venular resistance will increase capillary blood pressure as will a rise in mean venous pressure.

- *Plasma effective osmotic pressure*: This is a force that pulls water into a capillary and is measured in mm Hg. Plasma effective osmotic pressure (π_p) (Figure 14.2), also referred

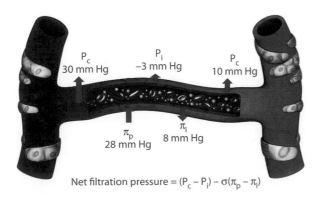

$$\text{Net filtration pressure} = (P_c - P_i) - \sigma(\pi_p - \pi_i)$$

Figure 14.2 Capillary with forces important for transcapillary exchange.

to as the oncotic pressure, is related mostly to the osmotic pressure of plasma proteins as follows:

	mm Hg
Albumin	20
Globulin	5
Fibrinogen	1

Notice that total osmotic pressure is not used here. Total osmotic pressure is attributable mostly to Na^+ and its associated anions and is close to 300 mosm/100 mL, which converts to over 5000 mm Hg. However, ions freely diffuse back and forth through the capillary wall, with accompanying water, and have no effect on net water movement. Ions are not normally "effective" in producing net movement of water as they freely move across the capillary wall.

Albumen has a small molecular size compared with the other plasma proteins, but it contributes the largest number of particles among the blood proteins. Osmotic pressure is strongly related to the number of insoluble particles in a liquid.

- *Interstitial fluid pressure*: Interstitial fluid pressure, P_i, normally is very low and in many areas of the body is below atmospheric pressure (Figure 14.2), such as in the lung and skin. P_i can increase when capillary permeability increases and produces tissue edema, such as in an allergic reaction or an insect bite. Interstitial fluid accumulation in the presence of lymphatic blockade is another example of increased interstitial fluid pressure.

- *Interstitial fluid effective osmotic pressure*: Interstitial fluid effective osmotic pressure, π_i (Figure 14.2), is related, in part, to plasma proteins that have leaked out of the capillary and into the interstitium. Interstitial space ground substance (hyaluronic acid, chondroitin SO_4, etc.) and compounds like lactate also contribute to π_i.

STARLING FORMULATION OF TRANSCAPILLARY FLUID MOVEMENT

- *Forces moving fluid out of a capillary*: Capillary blood pressure (P_c) is a force that pushes fluid out of a capillary into the interstitium (Figure 14.2). A simple analogy can be made to simple filtration, for instance, in making filter coffee. Pouring more water into the filter increases the fluid level above the filter membrane and enhances the drip rate.

  Interstitial fluid effective osmotic pressure (π_i) is a force that pulls fluid out of a capillary (Figure 14.2). This is because interstitial tissue proteins cannot cross into capillary blood. The tissue proteins occupy space that would otherwise be occupied by H_2O. This reduces water activity in the interstitium and draws water to it. A simple way of remembering this is that osmotic pressure is a sucking force that pulls water to it. π_i is normally a very small force.

  Negative interstitial fluid pressure (P_i) in, for instance, skin pulls water out of the capillary and into the interstitium (Figure 14.2). This is typically a very small magnitude force, but it does favor water movement out of a capillary. When P_i is positive it is a force moving water into a capillary.

- *Forces moving fluid into a capillary*: Plasma effective osmotic pressure (π_p) is, as noted above, a force related to plasma proteins, primarily albumin, which reduce plasma water activity. They reduce water activity because they cannot diffuse out of the capillary and take up space in the blood that would otherwise be occupied by H_2O. This force pulls H_2O into the capillary. Again, a simple way of remembering this is that this is a sucking force pulling water into the capillary from the interstitium.

If P_i is positive it will act to push fluid into a capillary and if arterial blood pressure is low enough, P_c can decrease enough to favor net movement of water into the capillary. **The effect of blood loss, low arterial blood pressure, and low Pc on transcapillary fluid exchange is presented in the self-study module The Pathophysiology of Hypovolemic Shock.**

- *Net fluid movement across a capillary wall*: The net fluid movement across a capillary wall is expressed as the net filtration pressure and is a balance of all four pushing and pulling forces that influence transcapillary exchange:

$$\text{Net Filtration Pressure} = (P_c - P_i) - \sigma(\pi_p - \pi_i)$$

This is a formula developed by Ernest Starling. Sigma (σ) is the reflection coefficient. If no albumin diffused through the capillary wall and escaped into the interstitium σ would equal 1.0. In other words, all the albumin trying to diffuse out of the capillary is "reflected" back into the capillary blood at the capillary wall. Proteins are large and have difficulty diffusing through a capillary wall and in most capillaries σ approximates 0.9.

Damage to capillaries due, for instance, to bacterial toxins and inflammation, can increase capillary permeability. Capillary permeability increases in an area of inflammation and σ decreases. Depending on the severity of the damage, water, electrolytes, proteins, and cells can diffuse out of damaged capillaries. This is seen, for instance, in vasogenic shock.

- *Change along a capillary*: There is resistance to flow in capillaries, but it is small as evidenced by the small fall in pressure as blood flows through a capillary (Figure 14.2). But there is enough resistance to result in P_c falling as blood flows from the arterial to venous end of a capillary (See Figure 11.6 in Chapter 11, Peripheral Circulation). Note in Figure 14.2 the fall in P_c along the length of the capillary. There can be subtle changes in π_p along the capillary length, not shown in Figure 14.2, but such changes are usually small. The net filtration pressure falls along a capillary as P_c falls and reabsorption predominates at the venous end of many capillaries. For instance, in Figure 14.2 consider the net filtration pressure (NFP) at the arteriolar and venous ends of the capillary:

$$\text{Arteriolar end NFP} = (30 - (-3)) - 0.9(28 - 8) = +15 \text{ mm Hg}$$
$$\text{Venous end NFP} = (10 - (-3)) - 0.9(28 - 2) = -5 \text{ mm Hg}$$

A negative net filtration pressure indicates a net movement of water into the capillary. In most capillary beds, there is a net loss of water, as there is here. Significant edema does not occur partly because the lymphatic system moves interstitial water back into the vascular compartment.

The self-study module Transcapillary Fluid Exchange: Starling Principle of Fluid Movement across a Capillary Wall contains clinical examples of edema formation and explanations of changes in net filtration pressure in clinical problems.

Also, there is an example of a change in net filtration pressure in a clinical problem presented in the self-study module The Pathophysiology of Hypovolemic Shock.

LYMPH AND LYMPHATICS

Normal lymph fluid is made up of capillary fluid transudate and large molecules including proteins and fats. Lymphatics begin as blind permeable endothelial sacs (blind sac = bag with only one opening) (Figures 14.1 and 14.3). Substances enter between the overlapping endothelial cells of the sac wall that act as flap valves (Figure 14.3). Larger lymphatic vessels have valves to ensure unidirectional flow toward the thorax (Figure 14.3). Most of the lymphatic flow collects into the thoracic duct, which empties into the left subclavian vein (Figure 14.3).

The lymphatic blind sac walls are made of endothelial cells that overlap and act like valves (Figure 14.3). Substances that diffuse into a sac move from the sac through the lymphatic vessels (Figure 14.3). Lymphatic fluid is propelled by at least two forces. Pulsations of smooth muscle in the lymphatic vessel walls in combination with valves (Figure 14.3) moves fluid forward. Also, the thoracic duct empties into the left subclavian vein, which is in the thorax. The subatmospheric pressure (suction) of the thorax facilitates lymph movement.

There are filaments attached to the sac endothelial cells (Figure 14.3). These anchoring filaments are attached to the surrounding interstitial structures. Tissue movement, such as limb movement and respiration, tugs on the filaments and pulls apart the overlapping endothelial cells allowing fluid and proteins, for instance, to enter the sacs.

Lymph flow rate is low and occurs primarily because of net fluid transudation from the capillary bed and uptake of the fluid by the lymphatics. Moving tissues, such as the lungs, gut, heart, and skeletal muscle, rhythmically squeeze lymphatics, which further facilitates fluid flow through the valves toward the thoracic duct. The flow rate is low, but total daily lymph flow is substantial and important for maintaining normal circulating blood volume. The brain has minimal lymphatic drainage.

DIFFUSION

Random movement of molecules and ions results in their eventual even dispersion throughout a solution. Whenever a concentration difference occurs, there is a net movement toward the area of lower concentration until equilibrium is restored.

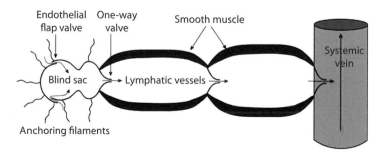

Figure 14.3 Lymphatic blind sac and lymphatic capillary structure. (From Levick JR. *An Introduction to Cardiovascular Physiology*, 5th ed. London, England: Hodder Arnold; 2011. With permission of Taylor and Francis Group.)

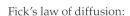

Fick's law of diffusion:

$$\frac{dn}{dt} = -DA\left(\frac{dc}{dx}\right)$$

where

t	= Time
n	= Amount of substance transported
D	= Free diffusion constant
A	= Transverse cross-sectional area of the tissue available for diffusion
(dc)/(dx)	= Concentration difference per unit distance

Each molecule or compound has a characteristic diffusion constant, D.

The radius of a substance or molecule must be small compared with pore size for diffusion through the capillary wall. Lipid soluble substances dissolve through the capillary wall.

Once across a capillary wall, molecules must diffuse through the interstitial space to reach cells. Fick's law of diffusion emphasizes the importance of concentration gradient, surface area, and distance for diffusion of a substance from and to the capillaries. For instance, working muscle consumes O_2 and muscle interstitial PO_2 decreases. PO_2 of blood entering the capillary is high. There is then a large dc/dx for O_2 from the blood to the muscle interstitium and muscle cell, and dn/dt is enhanced.

References for additional reading

Barrett KE et al. *Ganong's Review of Medical Physiology*, 23rd ed. New York: McGraw-Hill; 2010.

Boron WF. *Medical Physiology*, 2nd ed. Philadelphia: Elsevier; 2009.

Davis D. *Quick and Accurate 12-Lead ECG Interpretation*, 4th ed. Philadelphia: Elsevier; 2005.

Davis D. *Differential Diagnosis of Arrhythmia*, 2nd ed. Philadelphia: Elsevier; 1997.

Goldberger AL. *Clinical Electrocardiography*. 7th ed. Philadelphia: Mosby Elsevier; 2006, (16–18, p. 199).

Goldberger AL, Goldberger ZD, Shvilkin A. *Goldberger's Clinical Electrocardiography*, 9th ed. Philadelphia, PA: Elsevier; 2018.

Levick JR. *An Introduction to Cardiovascular Physiology*, 5th ed. London, England: Hodder Arnold; 2011.

Katz AM. *Physiology of the Heart*. 2nd ed. New York: Raven Press; 1992.

Malmivuo J, Plonsey R. *Bioelectromagnetism Principles and Applications of Bioelectric and Biomagnetic Fields*. 1995.

Rowell LB. *Human Circulation Regulation during Physical Stress*, Oxford: Oxford University Press; 1986.

Zipes DP, Jalife J. *Cardiac Electrophysiology from Bench to Bedside*. 6th ed. Philadelphia, PA: Elsevier; 2014.

Index

Absolute refractory period (ARP), 17–18

ACE, *see* Angiotensin converting enzyme

Acetylcholine (ACh), 21

ACh, *see* Acetylcholine

Acidic metabolites, 130

Acquired or congenital valvular heart disease, 78

ADH, *see* Antidiuretic hormone

Adult central nervous system, 123

Adverse remodeling, 120

Afterdepolarizations, 54, 55, 56

Afterload, 88–90; *see also* Ventricular function

Angiotensin converting enzyme (ACE), 110; *see also* Circulatory controls
    actions of, 112

Annulus fibrosus, 27

ANP, *see* Atrial natriuretic peptide

Antidiuretic hormone (ADH), 112

Aortic arch, 106

Aortic blood pressure
    exercise and, 99
    pulse and, 96

Aortic root, 74

Aortic stiffness, 96–97

Aortic valvular insufficiency, 78, 80

Aortic valvular regurgitation, *see* Aortic valvular insufficiency

ARP, *see* Absolute refractory period

Arrhythmia, 18
    atrial, 49–50
    Ca²⁺ influx, 54
    delayed afterdepolarizations, 56
    early afterdepolarizations, 55
    long QT syndrome, 56
    mechanisms of, 52–57
    reentry, 52–54
    respiratory sinus, 42–43
    Torsades de Pointes, 56, 57
    triggered activity, 54–55
    unidirectional block, 53

Arterial blood pressure, 95, 101, 119; *see also* Mean arterial blood pressure
    coronary vasculature perfusion, 52
    decrease in, 107
    mean, 95–99, 122
    regional characteristics of, 101

Arterial neural baroreceptors, 105; *see also* Circulatory controls
    aortic arch, 106
    carotid sinus, 105, 106–109
    structure, 105

Arterioles, 101, 117, 129, 135
    radius, 121–122
    vasodilation, 113

Arteriovenous anastomosis, *see* Metarterioles

Astrocytes, 123

Atrial arrhythmias, 49
    premature atrial beats, 49–50

Atrial fibrillation, 50–51

Atrial flutter, 50

Atrial myocytes, 11–12

Atrial natriuretic peptide (ANP), 112–113; *see also* Circulatory controls

Atrial premature beat, lower, 49–50

Atrial tachyarrhythmias, 18

Atrioventricular conduction blocks, 43
    dissociation, 45
    first degree, 43–45
    second degree, 44

Atrioventricular node (AV node), 12, 27; *see also* Cardiac electrical activity; Sinoatrial node
    latent pacemakers, 15
    refractory period, 18

Autonomic nervous system, 120; *see also* Circulatory controls

Autoregulation, 117–119; *see also* Circulatory controls
    in coronary vasculature, 127
    in resting skeletal muscle, 130

AV node, *see* Atrioventricular node

Baroreceptor, 105
    arterial neural, 105–109
    regions located at X's, 106
Beta adrenergic receptors, 129
Bipolar limb leads, 32–33
Blood–brain barrier, 124; *see also* Cerebral
      blood flow
Blood clotting and vascular endothelial
      factors, 114
Blood flow, 62–64; *see also* Circulation; Regional
      blood flow
    autoregulation of, 117–119
    capillary, 136, 137
    intermittent, 137
    laminar flow, 64
    local metabolic control of, 116–117
    siphon model, 63
    and temperature control, 133
    turbulent flow, 65
    types, 64–67
    velocity at cardiac output, 66
    velocity in circulation, 67
Blood pressure, 61; *see also* Circulation
    aortic pulse and, 96
    control, 105, 120
    high, 109
    at locations in circulation, 102
    measuring devices, 62
Blood viscosity, 64, 65
Blood volume distribution, 103
BNP, *see* Brain natriuretic peptide
Brain; *see also* Cerebral blood flow
    astrocytes, 123
    blood flow factors, 122
    metabolism, 124
    tumor, 123
Brain natriuretic peptide (BNP), 112–113; *see also*
      Circulatory controls
Bruit, 66
Bundle branch, 12–13
    blocks, 46
Bundle of HIS, 12–13, 27

Capillary, 135
    blood flow, 136, 137
    blood pressure, 137, 138
    transcapillary exchange, 137–138
    transcapillary fluid movement, 137, 138–140

Cardiac contractility, 85; *see also* Cardiac electrical
      activity; Cardiac muscle; Ventricular
      function
    drugs on, 87
    pressure-volume loop and, 87–88
    sympathetic stimulation of heart muscle, 86
    ventricular function curves, 85–87
Cardiac cycle, 71, 73
    atrial and ventricular phases of, 71
    atrial systole at end of diastole, 71
    coronary blood flow and, 127–128
    diastolic filling, 74–75
    ejection, 73–74
    events in left heart, 72
    intravascular pressures, 75
    isovolumetric contraction, 73
    isovolumetric relaxation, 74
    murmurs during, 78–81
    v wave, 75
Cardiac electrical activity, 9, 13; *see also* Ventricular
      myocyte electrophysiology
    atrial myocytes, 11–12
    atrioventricular node, 12
    bundle branches, 12–13
    bundle of HIS, 12–13
    Purkinje myocytes, 13
    sinoatrial node, 9–11
Cardiac muscle, 23; *see also* Cardiac contractility
    cell, 23
    desmosomes, 23
    gap junctions, 23, 24
    intercalated discs, 23
    sequential portions of, 4, 5
Cardiac muscle fiber, *see* Cardiac muscle—cell
Cardiac myocyte, *see* Cardiac muscle—cell
Cardiac output (CO), 64, 83
Cardiac valves, 71
Carotid sinus, 105; *see also* Arterial neural
      baroreceptors
    baroreceptor function, 106
    baroreceptor reflex response to arterial
      pressure, 107
    hemodynamic effects of posture change, 108
Carotid sinus, 105, 106–109
Cell cytoplasm, 3
Cerebral arteries, 121
Cerebral blood flow, 121; *see also* Circulation;
      Blood flow

arteriolar radius, 121–122

blood–brain barrier, 124

blood viscosity, 64, 65, 123

brain metabolism, 124

cerebral hypoxia, 122

changes in, 123

factors in brain blood flow, 122

intracranial pressure, 123

lymphatic drainage, 124

mean arterial pressure, 122

mean venous pressure, 122, 123, 137

regulation of, 121, 123

Cerebral hypoxia, 122

Chemoreceptors, 116; *see also* Circulatory controls

Circular movement, *see* Circus movement

Circulation, 59, 61, 71, 72; *see also* Blood flow;
    Microcirculation; Peripheral circulation

blood flow types, 64–67

blood pressure, 61

blood pressure measuring devices, 62

clinical significance, 67–69

energy, 61–62

flow, 62–64

pressure potential energy difference, 62

siphon model, 63

velocity, 67

Circulatory controls, 105

arterial blood pressure, 119

arterial neural baroreceptors, 105–109

autonomic nervous system, 120

autoregulation, 117–119

blood pressure control, 120

chemoreceptors, 116

heart failure, 120

hormonal controls, 109–116

local metabolic control, 116–117

salt and water metabolism, 119

veins in, 119

Circus movement, 54

CLBBB, *see* Complete left bundle branch block

Clotting, 116

CNP, *see* C-type natriuretic peptide

CO, *see* Cardiac output

Cold environment, exposure to, 133

Complete left bundle branch block (CLBBB),
    46–47, 48

Complete right bundle branch block
    (CRBBB), 46

Conduction; *see also* Ionic mechanisms,
    physiological consequences of

sequence in heart, 25

with sinus rhythm, normal, 42

system myocytes, 17

velocity, 16–17

Congenital valvular heart disease, 78

Contractility, 85–88

Coronary artery, 124–125

Coronary blood flow, 124; *see also* Blood flow

autoregulation, 127

and cardiac cycle, 127

clinical case, 128–129

control of, 126

coronary arteries, 124–125

diastole, 128

endothelial vasoactive factors, 128

myocardial oxygen consumption, 126–127

and oxygen supply, 125

sinus blood flow, 125

systole, 127

vasculature perfusion, 52

venous outflow, 128

work relationship, 126

Coronary sinus blood flow, 125

Coronary vasculature perfusion, 52

CRBBB, *see* Complete right bundle branch block

C-type natriuretic peptide (CNP), 112

Cutaneous blood flow, 132; *see also* Blood flow

and cold environment, 133

and temperature control, 133

and warm environment, 133–134

DBP, *see* Diastolic blood pressure

Depolarization, 5

of atrial or ventricular myocyte, 36

in horizontal plane, 42

vectors during atrial, 37

Desmosomes, 23

Diastole, 9, 78, 91, 128

Diastolic blood pressure (DBP), 108

Diastolic filling, 74–75

Diastolic murmur, 80–81

Dicrotic notch, 74

Diffusion, 140–141

Drugs, 55

action mechanism, 1

contractility, 87

Drugs (*Continued*)
    effects on ion channel function, 1
    in preventing reentry, 54
    in prolonging myocardial action potentials, 57
    side effect, 1
Dynamic exercise, 90, 99
Dysfunctional endothelium, 115; *see also*
        Circulatory controls
    abnormal endothelial cell function, 115
    endothelins, 115
    thromboxane, 116

ECG, *see* Electrocardiogram
EDHF, *see* Endothelium-derived hyperpolarizing
        factors
EDV, *see* End-diastolic volume
EF, *see* Ejection fraction
Einthoven's triangle, 38
Ejection fraction (EF), 91
Electrical activation sequence in heart, 26
Electrical activity in heart, 25
    annulus fibrosus, 27
    atrioventricular node, 27
    bundle of His, 27
    conduction sequence in heart, 25
    conduction system myocytes, 17
    gap junction function, 25
    sequence of, 26
    ventricular conducting system, 27
Electrocardiogram (ECG), 29
    abnormal ventricular beats, 51
    atrial arrhythmias, 49–50
    atrial fibrillation, 50–51
    atrial flutter, 50
    atrioventricular and intraventricular
        conduction blocks, 43
    bipolar limb leads, 32–33
    bundle branch blocks, 46
    CLBBB, 46–47, 48
    complete heart block, 45
    CRBBB, 46
    first degree atrioventricular block, 43–44
    frontal and horizontal planes, 32
    frontal plane leads, 31
    frontal plane vectors, 35–40
    horizontal plane leads, 34
    lead aVF lead and axis, 34
    lead aVL lead and axis, 33

    lead aVR lead and axis, 33
    mean electrical axis, 41
    mechanisms of arrhythmias, 52–57
    monitoring leads, 35
    normal conduction with normal sinus rhythm, 42
    patterns of abnormal rhythms, 49–52
    patterns of heart conduction, 42–49
    precordial leads, 35, 41–42
    precordial leads and V1 and V6 ventricular
        complexes, 41
    P wave, 30
    QRS complex, 30
    QT interval, 31
    respiratory sinus arrhythmia, 42–43
    second degree atrioventricular block, 44–45
    signal, 29
    standard lead system, 31–35
    ST segment, 31
    T wave, 30, 31
    unipolar limb lead, 33
    ventricular depolarization, 42
    ventricular fibrillation, 52
    ventricular premature beats, 51
    ventricular tachycardia, 51–52
    waves, 30–31
    Wolff–Parkinson–White, 47–49
End-diastolic volume (EDV), 91
Endothelial cell, 113
    dysfunctional, 115–116
    junctions, 124
Endothelial vasoactive factors, 128
Endothelins, 115
Endothelium-derived hyperpolarizing factors
        (EDHF), 114
End-systolic pressure volume relationship
        (ESPVR), 85
ESPVR, *see* End-systolic pressure volume
        relationship
Exercise and aortic blood pressure, 99

Feedback mechanisms, 59
First heart sound, 75
Fourth heart sound, 78
Frank–Starling law of the heart, 83, 84; *see also*
        Ventricular function
Frontal plane vectors, 35; *see also* Mean vector
    during atrial depolarization, 37
    myocyte depolarization, 36

Gap junctions, 23, 24
    function, 25
Gastrointestinal blood flow, 132; *see also*
        Blood flow

Heart; *see also* Circulatory controls
    complete block, 45
    conduction patterns, 42–49
    failure, 120
    in vivo control of, 93
    sympathetic stimulation of muscle, 86
Heart rate control, 21
    parasympathetic activity, 21
    SA node action potential simulation, 22
    sympathetic activity, 21–22
Heart sounds, 75
    first, 75
    fourth, 78
    second, 76–77
    third, 77, 78
    transmural pressure, 76
High blood pressure, 109
Hormonal control of circulation, 109; *see also*
        Circulatory controls
    antidiuretic hormone, 112
    atrial and brain natriuretic peptides, 112–113
    clotting, 116
    dysfunctional endothelium, 115–116
    renin-angiotensin-aldosterone system,
        109–112
    vascular endothelial factors, 113–115
Hydrostatic pressure, *see* Capillary—blood
        pressure
Hypertension, *see* High blood pressure

Incisura, *see* Dicrotic notch
Intercalated discs, 23
Intermittent blood flow, 137
Interstitial fluid effective osmotic pressure, 138
Intracranial pressure, 123
Intravascular pressures, normal, 75
Ionic mechanisms, physiological consequences
        of, 15
    conduction velocity, 16–17
    K^+ effect on transmembrane potential, 19
    latent pacemakers, 15
    pacemaker hierarchy, 15
    refractory period, 17–18

Ions
    in cell cytoplasm, 3
    movement in gap junctions, 24, 25
Isovolumetric contraction, 73
Isovolumetric relaxation, 74

Juxtaglomerular cells, 110

LA, *see* Left arm; Left atrium
Laminar flow, 64; *see also* Blood flow
Latent pacemakers, 15; *see also* Ionic mechanisms,
        physiological consequences of
Left arm (LA), 38
Left atrium (LA), 71
Left leg (LL), 38
Left ventricle (LV), 41, 71
LL, *see* Left leg
Local metabolic control, 116–117; *see also*
        Circulatory controls
Long QT syndrome, 56
LV, *see* Left ventricle
Lymphatic blind sac, 140
Lymphatic capillary structure, 140
Lymphatic drainage, 124
Lymph flow rate, 140
Lymph fluid, 140

Maximal diastolic potential (MDP), 9
MBP, *see* Mean arterial blood pressure
MDP, *see* Maximal diastolic potential
Mean aortic blood pressure, 95; *see also* Peripheral
        circulation
Mean arterial blood pressure (MBP), 108
Mean vector, 37; *see also* Frontal plane vectors
    for atrial depolarization and Einthoven's
        triangle, 38
    with depolarized ventricular myocytes, 40
    for ventricular septal depolarization, 39
Mean venous pressure, 122, 123, 137
Metabolic control of circulation, 116–117
Metarterioles, 135–136
Microcirculation, 135; *see also* Blood flow;
        Circulation
    arterioles, 135
    capillaries, 135
    capillary blood flow, 136, 137
    diffusion, 140–141
    intermittent blood flow, 137

Microcirculation (*Continued*)
    lymphatic blind sac and lymphatic capillary
        structure, 140
    and lymphatics, 136, 140
    metarterioles, 135–136
    microcirculation and lymphatics, 136
    nature of blood flow in, 136
    net filtration pressure, 139
    postcapillary resistance, 136
    starling formulation of transcapillary fluid
        movement, 138–140
    transcapillary exchange, 137–138
    transcapillary fluid movement, 137
Monitoring leads, 35
Moving tissues, 140
Murmur, 78; *see also* Cardiac cycle
    diastolic, 80–81
    systolic, 79–80
Myocardial muscle fiber, *see* Cardiac muscle—cell
Myocardial myocyte, *see* Cardiac muscle—cell
Myocardial oxygen consumption determinants,
    126–127
Myocardial resting force, 92
Myocardium, primate ventricular, 92
Myocyte, 25
Myoplasmic Ca^{2+} overload, 54

Na^+/Ca^{2+} exchange (NCX), 11
Natriuretic peptides, 112–113
NCX, *see* Na^+/Ca^{2+} exchange
Negative interstitial fluid pressure, 138
Neprilysin, 113
Net filtration pressure (NFP), 139
Neural reflexes, 105
NFP, *see* Net filtration pressure
Nitric oxide (NO), 113–114
NO, *see* Nitric oxide
Noise, *see* Murmur
Norepinephrine, 21
Normal intravascular pressures in people, 75
Normal sinus rhythm, 15

PA, *see* Pulmonary artery
Pacemaker
    hierarchy, 15
    latent, 15
    potential, 9, 10
PAI-1, *see* Plasminogen-activator inhibitor type 1

Parasympathetic activity, 21
Parasympathetic nerve action potentials, 101
Peripheral arteriolar vasodilation, 113
Peripheral circulation, 95; *see also* Circulation
    aortic pulse and blood pressure, 96
    aortic stiffness, 96–97
    blood volume distribution, 103
    exercise and aortic blood pressure, 99
    mean arterial pressure, 95–99
    pulse pressure, 95–99
    relationship of pressure, flow, and
        resistance, 97
    resistance, 100–103
    responses to vascular resistance, 100
Peripheral runoff, 95
Plasma effective osmotic pressure, 137, 138–139
Plasminogen-activator inhibitor type 1 (PAI-1), 115
Poiseuille's law, 100, 117; *see also* Pulse pressure;
    Resistance
    variables in, 101
Postcapillary resistance, 136
Precordial leads, 35, 41–42
Preexcitation, *see* Wolff–Parkinson–White
Preload, 83–85
Premature atrial beats, 49–50
Pressoreceptor, *see* Baroreceptor
Pressure, 61
    receptor, *see* Baroreceptor
    -volume loop, 84–85
    -volume relation, 91–93
Primate ventricular myocardium, 92
Prostacyclin, 114
Pulmonary artery (PA), 71
Pulmonary blood flow, 130; *see also* Blood flow
    characteristics, 130–131
    posture and exercise effect, 131–132
Pulse pressure, 95–99; *see also* Peripheral
    circulation; Poiseuille's law
    changes in, 98–100
    determinants of, 97–98
    mean arterial pressure and, 95–96
Purkinje myocytes, 13
    cardiac electrical activity, 13
    latent pacemakers, 15
P wave, 30

QRS complex, 30
QT interval, 31

RA, *see* Right arm; Right atrium

RAAS, *see* Renin-angiotensin-aldosterone system

RBCs, *see* Red blood cells

RBF, *see* Renal blood flow

Rectification, 6

Red blood cells (RBCs), 101, 136

Reentry, 18

Refractory period, 17; *see also* Ionic mechanisms, physiological consequences of
    absolute, 17–18
    reentry, 18
    relative, 18
    SA and AV node, 18
    ventricular and conduction system myocytes, 17

Regional blood flow, 121; *see also* Blood flow
    cerebral blood flow, 121–124
    coronary blood flow, 124–129
    cutaneous blood flow, 132–134
    gastrointestinal blood flow, 132
    pulmonary blood flow, 130–132
    renal blood flow, 132
    skeletal muscle blood flow, 129–130

Regurgitation, *see* Valvular insufficiency

Relative refractory period (RRP), 18

Renal blood flow (RBF), 132; *see also* Blood flow

Renin, 110
    actions of, 112

Renin-angiotensin-aldosterone system (RAAS), 109–112

Repolarization of ventricles, 40

Resistance to flow, 100; *see also* Peripheral circulation
    in vivo resistances, 103
    mean blood pressure at locations in circulation, 102
    parallel vascular resistance, 102
    Poiseuille's law, 100–101
    regional characteristics of arterial blood pressure, 101
    series vascular resistance, 102
    single resistance, 103
    three parallel resistances, 103
    two series resistances, 103
    vascular conductance, 102–103

Respiratory sinus arrhythmia, 42–43

Rhythm patterns, abnormal, 49–52

Right arm (RA), 38

Right atrium (RA), 71

Right ventricle (RV), 41, 71

RRP, *see* Relative refractory period

RV, *see* Right ventricle

Salt and water metabolism, 119

SA node, *see* Sinoatrial node

Sarcolemma, charge separation by, 3

Sarcoplasmic reticulum (SR), 11

SBP, *see* Systolic blood pressure

Second heart sound, 76–77

Sigma, 139

Single resistance, 103

Sinoatrial node (SA node), 9; *see also* Cardiac electrical activity
    action potential, 10, 22
    normal sinus rhythm, 15
    pacemaker potential, 9, 10, 15
    phase 0 upstroke, 9
    phase 1 and phase 2, 10
    phase 3, 10
    phase 4, 11
    refractory period, 18
    repolarization, 10
    sympathetic stimulation of, 21

Sinus rhythm, normal, 15

Siphon model, 63; *see also* Circulation

Skeletal muscle blood flow, 129; *see also* Blood flow
    anatomical and mechanical considerations, 129
    autoregulation, 130
    control, 129
    oxygen delivery, 130
    sympathetic effects, 129

Skeletal muscle pump, 84

SR, *see* Sarcoplasmic reticulum

Standard lead system, 31–35

Starling formulation of transcapillary fluid movement, 138–140

Stiffness, 95

Streamlined flow, *see* Laminar flow

Stroke volume (SV), 83, 84, 91

ST segment, 31

SV, *see* Stroke volume

Sympathetic activity, 21–22

Sympathetic nervous system, 119, 121

Sympathetic stimulation of heart muscle, 86

Systole, 71, 78, 127

Systolic blood pressure (SBP), 108
Systolic murmur, 79–80

Temperature control, 133
Thoroughfare channel, *see* Metarterioles
Thromboxane, 116
Tissue plasminogen activator (t-PA), 115
Torsades de Pointes, 56, 57
t-PA, *see* Tissue plasminogen activator
Transcapillary exchange, 137–138
Transcapillary fluid movement, 137
    starling formulation of, 138–140
Transmural pressure, 76, 131
Tumor, brain, 123
Turbulent flow, 65; *see also* Blood flow
T wave, 30, 31

Unidirectional block, 53
Unipolar limb lead, 33

Valvular heart disease, 78
Valvular insufficiency, 78, 80
Valvular stenosis, 78
Vascular conductance, 102–103
Vascular endothelial factors, 113; *see also*
        Circulatory controls
    effects on blood clotting, 114
    endothelium-derived hyperpolarizing
        factors, 114
    nitric oxide, 113–114
    prostacyclin, 114
Vascular resistance, 102
    three parallel resistances, 103
    two series resistances, 103
Vasodilators, 116; *see also* Vascular endothelial factors
Vasopressin, *see* Antidiuretic hormone
Vectors during atrial depolarization, 37
Veins, 119; *see also* Circulatory controls
Venous outflow, 128
Venous pressure, mean, 122, 123, 137
Ventricular beats, abnormal, 51
Ventricular complexes, V1 and V6, 41
Ventricular conducting system, 27; *see also*
        Electrical activity in heart
Ventricular depolarization in horizontal plane, 42
Ventricular fibrillation, 52

Ventricular filling, 83–84; *see also* Ventricular
        function
Ventricular function, 83, 85–87
    afterload, 88–90
    changes in, 90–91
    changes in posture, 91
    changes in ventricular filling, 83–84
    contractility, 85–88
    control of heart *in vivo*, 93
    curves, 85–87
    ejection fraction, 91
    exercise, 90–91
    Frank–Starling law of the heart, 83, 84
    myocardial resting force, 92
    passive pressure-volume relation, 91–93
    passive/resting ventricular pressure-volume
        relation, 92
    preload, 83–85
    pressure-volume loop, 84–85
    primate ventricular myocardium, 92
Ventricular muscle cell action potential, 5
    adequate, 5
    negative current, 5
    phase 0, 5–6
    phase 1, 6, 8
    phase 2, 6–7
    phase 3, 7–8
    plateau portion of, 7
    rectification, 6
Ventricular myocyte electrophysiology, 3; *see also*
        Cardiac electrical activity
    action potential, 5–8
    charge separation by sarcolemma, 3
    negative ions, 3
    resting potential, 3–4
    ventricular action potential and ionic
        currents, 4
Ventricular premature beats, 51
Ventricular pressure, 91
Ventricular septal depolarization, 39
Ventricular tachycardia, 51–52
Venules, 135, 136; *see also* Arterioles
v wave, 75; *see also* Cardiac cycle

Warm environment, exposure to, 133–134
Wolff–Parkinson–White (WPW), 47–49